Noncompaction Cardiom

Kadir Caliskan • Osama I. Soliman
Folkert J. ten Cate
Editors

Noncompaction Cardiomyopathy

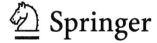

Springer

Editors
Kadir Caliskan
Erasmus MC University Medical Center
Department of Cardiology
Rotterdam
The Netherlands

Osama I. Soliman
Erasmus MC University Medical Center
The Thoraxcenter
Rotterdam
The Netherlands

Folkert J. ten Cate
Erasmus MC University Medical Center
Department of Cardiology
Rotterdam
The Netherlands

ISBN 978-3-030-17722-5   ISBN 978-3-030-17720-1   (eBook)
https://doi.org/10.1007/978-3-030-17720-1

This Springer imprint is published by the registered company Springer Nature Switzerland AG
The registered company address is: Gewerbestrasse 11, 6330 Cham, Switzerland

Preface

Why Do We Need This book?

Noncompaction of the left ventricle or *noncompaction cardiomyopathy* (*NCCM*) is a new clinic-pathological entity that was first described by Rolf Engberding et al. in 1984 as an isolated case with this abnormal myocardial pattern with the "persistence of isolated myocardial sinusoids". It is characterized by a prominent trabecular meshwork and deep intertrabecular recesses communicating with the left ventricular (LV) cavity, morphologically reminiscent of early cardiac development, and is therefore thought to be caused by an arrest of normal embryogenesis of the myocardium. We are therefore proud and very grateful for Dr. Engberding's excellent contribution for the first chapter of this title.

The initial presentation includes congestive heart failure, thromboembolic events, and (potentially lethal) arrhythmias, including sudden cardiac death. NCCM may be a part of a more generalized cardiomyopathy, involving both the morphologically normal and the predominantly apical abnormal LV segments. The cardiological features of NCCM range from asymptomatic, isolated forms in adults to severe congenital, pediatric abnormalities.

NCCM may be isolated or non-isolated, i.e hereditary and appears to be genetically heterogeneous. The majority of NCCM diagnosed in adults is isolated. Non-isolated forms of NCCM are more frequent in childhood and may co-occur with congenital heart malformations or may be part of complex genetic or chromosomal syndrome. An important proportion of isolated NCCM in children and adults has been associated with mutations in the same *sarcomere* genes that are involved in hypertrophic (HCM), dilated (DCM), and restrictive cardiomyopathy (RCM). The absence of a genetic defect does not preclude a genetic cause of NCCM. In approximately half of the familial NCCM, the genetic defect remains unknown. The shared sarcomere defects and the occurrence of HCM and DCM in families with NCCM patients indicate that at least some forms of NCCM are part of a broader cardiomyopathy spectrum. Furthermore, the combination of NCCM and neuromuscular disorders is observed in adults as well as in children.

Increased awareness of this disease entity made us recognize more and more cases of NCCM, especially with the help of modern cardiac imaging modalities like contrast echocardiography, Ct-scan and MRI, allowing better visualization of the ventricular cavities, endocardial delineation, and myocardial walls. However, in daily clinical practice, many questions about several clinical aspects remained open, because the available literature consists mainly of case reports and case series. The prevalence of NCCM is largely unknown, and many demographic and epidemiologic questions remain yet to be elucidated. Furthurmore, prevention and appropriate risk stratification of sudden cardiac death remain highly challenging. Strategies to improve the outcome of patients with this rare disease come from large case series but really need multicentre registry-based studies to expand, confirm, and refine findings.

This title is written by a panel of experts, who have been not only daily involved with this new clinical entity but have also proven academic track record with this yet rare clinical entity. It will provide a comprehensive but concise overview of non-compaction cardiomyopathy and will be the first ever reference book for clinicians in the field of cardiology, electrophysiology, internal medicine, and clinical and molecular genetics, paediatricians, pathologists, neurologists, and, last but not least, general practitioners involved in daily basis in the care and cure of these patients.

This book will include 10 chapters, about 167 pages, depicted in the Table of Contents. Key messages are highlighted at the end of each chapter. We expect that this work will be interesting and helpful to a wide range of readers, clinicians and scientist, and ultimately have a positive impact on the daily care of these patients.

Rotterdam, The Netherlands   Kadir Caliskan
Rotterdam, The Netherlands   Osama I. Soliman
Rotterdam, The Netherlands   Folkert J. ten Cate

Contents

Noncompaction Cardiomyopathy, a Novel Clinical Entity (Historical Perspective)

Rolf Engberding and Birgit Gerecke

Introduction

Better understanding and increased awareness of a newly detected morphologic abnormality or disease entity is mostly connected to the progress in adequate imaging modalities.

The diagnosis of a spongy, apparently embryonic myocardial morphology has initially been shown only in newborns and infants on necropsy findings and later on angiographic results. But the breakthrough in the ante mortem diagnosis and the awareness of the disease began with the first description of the echocardiographic diagnosis of this abnormal myocardial pattern by one of the authors (R.E.) (Fig. 1.1) [1].

Further improvement in cardiovascular imaging quality, including modern echo-, MRI- and CT- modalities, has tremendously increased the numbers of detected cases with this myocardial pattern, even, in apparently healthy persons, thus, enforcing the need for improved diagnostic criteria to prevent mis- or over-diagnosis with its potential adverse consequences.

But the current concepts in diagnosis and management of a disease cannot be understood completely without a review of the historical background, which will be subsequently presented for this cardiac anomaly.

R. Engberding (✉)
Internal Medicine and Cardiology, amO MVZ Wolfsburg, Wolfsburg, Germany

B. Gerecke
Clinic for Cardiology and Pneumology, University Medical Center Göttingen, Göttingen, Germany

© Springer Nature Switzerland AG 2019
K. Caliskan et al. (eds.), *Noncompaction Cardiomyopathy*,
https://doi.org/10.1007/978-3-030-17720-1_1

Fig. 1.1 Echocardiography of the first published patient with isolated left ventricular noncompaction. Apical long axis view. *LV* left ventricle, *LA* left atrium, *AO* aorta. Arrows mark huge and deep spaces within the left ventricular wall

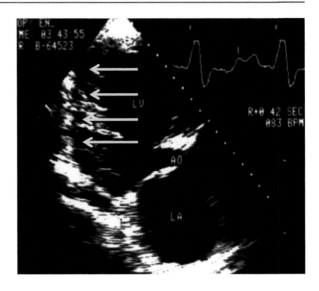

History

Due to the high systolic intraventricular pressure in case of atretic semilunar valve with intact ventricular septum, intramyocardial diverticula and sinusoids have been early observed and have been considered representing persistence and ectasia of the embryonic intertrabecular spaces and their communication with the coronary system [2–4]. In 1964, Lauer et al. observed 2 of 4 cases with pulmonary valve atresia and intact ventricular septum with sinusoids ending blindly in the myocardium. Additionally, they discussed, that during normal embryogenesis of the myocardium primarily a loose cellular epimyocardial meshwork develops, which, subsequently, becomes more compact, especially towards the epicardial surface, with intertrabecular spaces evolving [4].

In 1969, Feldt et al. reported on the clinical, angiographic and autopsy findings in a 3 months old girl with intractable congestive heart failure due to cyanotic congenital heart disease. The autopsy revealed a complete situs inversus, a muscular subpulmonic stenosis, a common atrioventricular valve lying above a ventricular septal defect and a common atrium. The wall of both ventricles showed a two layered myocardial structure with a thick spongy inner layer and a compact outer layer. Feldt et al. called this observation "anomalous ventricular myocardial patterns in a child with complex congenital heart disease" [5].

It was in 1984, that the first case of an adult patient with this anomalous ventricular myocardial pattern in absence of other structural malformations of the heart has been described, including its echocardiographic appearance [1]. In this early publication, the myocardial pattern of the disease was referred to as "persistence of isolated myocardial sinusoids" recognizing the persistence of embryonic myocardial morphology found in the absence of other cardiac anomalies. In a subsequent publication, Jenni et al. confirmed the initial observation, that the persistence of embryonic morphology of the myocardium can occur as an isolated disease, and they used the same terminology [6].

In 1990, Chin et al. proposed the term "isolated noncompaction of left ventricular myocardium" assuming that this disease was due to an arrest of the normal compaction process during endomyocardial morphogenesis, what, interestingly, Feldt et al. had already suggested in the report on their non-isolated case [7]. Chin et al. reported on 8 cases with isolated left ventricular noncompaction, 1 adult and 7 children, demonstrating the necropsy findings in 3 of them. Their histological results of the affected myocardium resembled the earlier findings of Dusek et al. that the intertrabecular recesses were covered with endothelium in continuity with the ventricular endothelium [8]. This observation was one reason to conclude, that the term "isolated noncompaction of left ventricular myocardium" should be more appropriate than "persisting isolated myocardial sinusoids" [1, 7].

An overview on the historical perspective is presented in Fig. 1.2.

Myocardial Development

The development of the heart involves wondrous and precisely regulated molecular and embryogenetic events [9, 10]. These events, triggered by specific signaling molecules and mediated by tissue-specific transcription factors, are highly complex. The cellular components that give rise to the myocardium have multiple origins, and de novo addition of myocardial cells to the developing heart occurs at various points during embryogenesis, initially from the primary heart field, and later from the secondary heart field [11]. The myocardial development includes the formation of 2 different myocardial layers within the ventricular wall, i.e., the trabecular layer and the subepicardial compact layer [12–14]. Due to observations in several studies, the process of ventricular trabeculation was considered to start in gestational week 12, when protrusions of the endocardial layer develop into myocardial trabeculations, thus creating an increased surface for the demanding blood supply of the rapidly growing myocardium prior to the development of the coronary circulation [15, 16]. As result of this process, the embryonic myocardium consists of a sponge-like meshwork of interwoven myocardial fibers forming trabeculae with intertrabecular recesses, which communicate with the left ventricular cavity [12–14]. The process of cardiac trabeculation is dependent on endocardial-myocardial interactions involving secretion of various factors such as neuregulin, serotonin 2B receptor, vascular endothelial growth factor and angiopoietin-1 [9, 10]. A lot of evidence exists, that these processes and protein expressions underlie a complex genetic regulation. Interestingly, it has been shown, that different specific genes are necessary for the growth of each, the right and the left ventricle and that these genes are expressed in the ventricular trabeculations but not within the interventricular septum [17, 18].

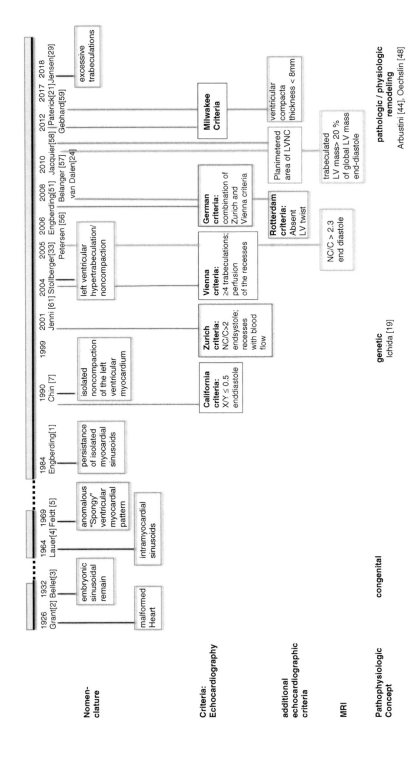

Fig. 1.2 Historical overview of left ventricular noncompaction: important landmarks of nomenclature, diagnostic criteria and pathophysiologic concepts

In the next stage of heart development, the ventricular myocardium was assumed to undergo gradual compaction, which usually should be completed by the end of gestational week 16 [15, 16]. The compaction process should be accompanied by further myocardial growth and increasing intracardial pressure, leading to compression of the relatively large intertrabecular spaces to capillaries, while large spaces within the trabecular meshwork gradually flatten or disappear [12–14, 19]. Concomitantly, the rearrangement of the myocardial blood supply includes the formation of coronary veins, which precede the coronary arteries in the development and which initially communicate with the embryonic terminal blood bed, in terms of intertrabecular spaces and sinusoids [8]. At the end of the cardiac developmental process, the coronary circulation should be completely established, providing the whole blood supply of the myocardium. At this point, usually no vascular communications between the former intertrabecular spaces and the coronary vascular or capillary system should remain [8, 19, 20].

The compaction process of the ventricular myocardium was suggested to normally progress from the epicardium to endocardium and from the base of the heart towards the apex [8, 19–22]. Thus, due to this assumption, in case of left ventricular noncompaction it can be supposed, that the left ventricular apex may be always affected. First clinical data support this suggestion [23].

During the process of increasing myocardial growth, the spiral patterns of cardiomyocytes seem to develop, leading to obliquely oriented myocardial fibers, varying from smaller radius and right-handed helix at the subendocardium to a larger radius and left-handed helix at the subepicardium. Thus, as functional consequence of the left ventricular myocardium, a clockwise basal rotation occurs, followed by a counterclockwise apical rotation, resulting in a cyclic systolic left ventricular twist. Interestingly, some clinical data suggest, that in cases of left ventricular noncompaction no systolic twisting deformation of the left ventricle is present, leading to the conclusion, that in these cases the spiral pattern of cardiomyocytes has not been developed properly [20, 24, 25].

Since the assumption of a compaction process following the phase of embryonic myocardial trabeculation during normal cardiac development has been widely accepted, at least since the publication of Chin et al. [7] up to now, observations of recent studies may allow new insights into the normal embryonic development of the heart. How far this may also alter our understanding of the etiology and pathophysiology of left ventricular noncompaction, has to be shown by the results of further research. The new data suggests, that from the very early phase of heart development around week 4, the growing ventricles start to acquire trabeculations, which are increasing within days to spongy formations. By gestational week 6 in human, the trabeculations have effectively ceased to proliferate, whereas the compact myocardium continues to grow, resulting in an exterior expansion of the ventricles as well in the development of ventricular lumina [17, 26–32].

Left Ventricular Noncompaction/Noncompaction Cardiomyopathy: Changes in Nomenclature—Uncertainties in Etiology

Changes in nomenclature often reflect the alterations in the actual knowledge of a disease. Regarding this topic, it ranges from the description of a "spongy myocardial pattern" over the term "persistence of isolated myocardial sinusoids", to the terms "left ventricular noncompaction (LVNC) or noncompaction cardiomyopathy (NCCM)" and "left ventricular hypertrabeculation (LVHT)" [1, 2, 6, 7, 33].

LVNC or NCCM has early been controversely considered a "primary genetic cardiomyopathy" as classified by the American Heart Association and an "unclassified cardiomyopathy" as proposed by the European Society of Cardiology [34, 35]. The classification of the American Heart Association has taken into account, that NCCM was considered to occur due to a genetically determined failure of the myocardial compaction process during normal development of the heart. This decision was based on the results of increasing numbers of studies showing, that mutations of various, especially sarcomeric genes, involved in the normal cardiac morphogenesis, can be observed in cases of NCCM [14, 21, 36].

Detailed data of the genetic involvement in this disease are presented in Chap. 8.

Nevertheless, other pathogenetic processes than failure in the genetic regulation of the cardiac developmental process have also been discussed, and various cases with an acquired form of this abnormal myocardial pattern have been published [37]. Especially, in athletes performing vigorous training and in pregnant women, an acquired development of the myocardial pattern of an increased or excessive trabecular morphology could be observed, which obviously was due to different conditions of ventricular volume or pressure load in these cases (Fig. 1.3) [38–41].

As mentioned earlier, the younger past brought up some important new studies with fundamentally different results regarding the developing and trabecular growing of the normal embryonic myocardium leading to different conclusions, especially to the assumption, that no real compaction process may be present in the normal cardiac development [29, 42, 43]. In case of NCCM Jensen et al. found, that the excessive trabeculations did not have the identity of the normal embryonic trabeculations [29]. Based on these observations, they suggested, that noncompaction may not be the result of a failure in a compaction process but instead results from the compacted myocardium of the ventricular wall, growing into the ventricular lumen in a trabecular fashion [29]. Consequently, it seems, that the term "LVHT" may be more appropriate than "LVNC".

The terms "LVNC" and "LVHT" are clearly descriptive, characterizing a typical ventricular wall anatomy but not a specific functional profile. Thus, these terms may not be necessarily used as synonyms for a cardiomyopathy [44]. This assumption is obviously supported by the observations of Jensen et al. and the conclusions of Anderson et al., who introduced the term "excessive trabeculations", describing

Fig. 1.3 Echocardiography of a young male athlete (diagnosis by chance). Left ventricle in the apical 4-chamber view. The arrows mark increased prominent apical trabeculations

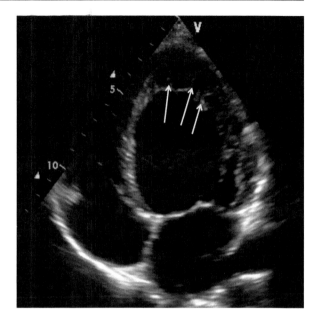

rather a myocardial phenotype of unknown origin or a kind of bystander in the presence of additional cardiac lesions than a cardiomyopathy [29, 42].

Left Ventricular Noncompaction: Phenotype or Established Cardiomyopathy?

Primarily, LVNC described a typical myocardial pattern on echocardiography with a subepicardially located compacted layer and a subendocardial noncompacted layer, which should be at least twice as thick as the compacted layer, presenting with increased, at least 4 prominent left ventricular trabeculations and deep intertrabecular recesses [33, 45]. But a lot of data have been published, that the current diagnostic criteria are not specific enough to safely prevent mis- or over-diagnosis of this disease [46, 47].

Consequently, it is debated, if LVNC should be considered rather a phenotype than an established cardiomyopathy; and when it is a phenotype, is it the result of a physiologic or pathologic remodeling of the myocardium [47, 48]? A very new multicenter study enhances the role of genetic testing in distinguishing genetic determined NCCM from the non-genetic phenotype LVNC [49]. Based on these important results, it can be suggested, that it might be possible in the future to distinguish a healthy person, e.g., an athlete, with the phenotype of LVNC due to a physiologic reversible remodeling of the myocardium from an asymptomatic

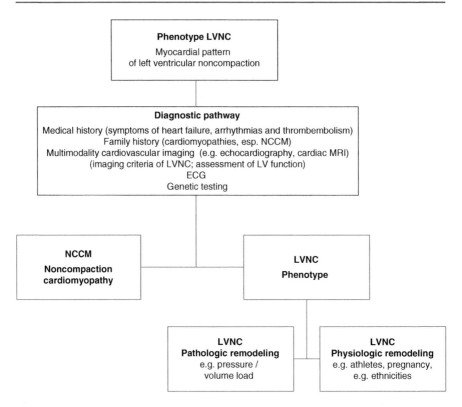

Fig. 1.4 Left ventricular noncompaction: phenotype (LVNC) and cardiomyopathy (NCCM), modified from [48]

NCCM. Additionally in this differentiation, the phenotype with pathologic myocardial remodeling due to volume or pressure overload or in conjunction with other cardiomyopathies, such as dilated or hypertrophic cardiomyopathy, has also to be considered.

According to the advanced suggestions of Oechslin and Jenni [48] regarding their clearly structured flow chart "from the myocardial phenotype of LVNC to NCCM", some minor modification might facilitate the terminology (Fig. 1.4).

Until a uniformly accepted clear distinction between LVNC and NCCM is available for clinical use, e.g., achieved by genetic testing or advanced cardiac imaging criteria, it may be proposed to consider NCCM, when isolated LVNC with systolic/diastolic left ventricular dysfunction and/or abnormal ECG findings and/or symptoms of heart failure, supraventricular or ventricular arrhythmias, collapse, syncope and/or thrombembolism and/or a family history of NCCM is present.

Clinical Entity of the First Published Case with Isolated NCCM

The first published case with isolated NCCM was a 33 year old woman. As her history revealed, she first presented to her family doctor at the age of 15 years with palpitations. At this time an ECG was performed, revealing a complete left bundle branch block. Other personal history findings were: diphtheria at the age of 2 years, recurrent tonsillitis and pneumonia in childhood, tonsillectomy at 7 years of age. The family history was unremarkable. When she sought medical help at the age of 33 years, she complained of palpitations and exertional dyspnea. A short systolic murmur was present over the apex. Otherwise, physical examination was normal, especially no physical signs of heart failure were found.

On chest x-ray, the heart was large and the pulmonary veins were congested. The ECG revealed complete left bundle branch block (QRSd 190 ms), prolonged PR interval (240 ms) and ventricular ectopic beats and couplets, which might have been the reason for the complaints of palpitations.

The 2-D-echocardiogram showed left ventricular enlargement and wall thickening, while right heart dimensions were normal. Within the left ventricular myocardium of all wall segments including the left ventricular apex, huge and deep spaces could be observed (Fig. 1.5).

The huge spaces within the left ventricular wall communicated with the left ventricular cavity but not with the coronary arteries as could be observed by additional coronary and left ventricular angiography (Fig. 1.6) [1].

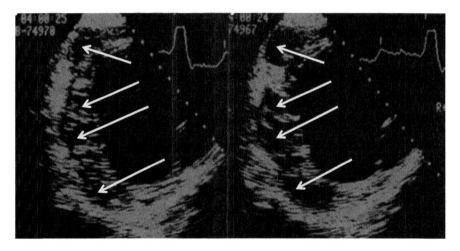

Fig. 1.5 Echocardiography of the first published patient with isolated left ventricular noncompaction. Parasternal short axis view at endsystole (left) and enddiastole. Huge and deep spaces (arrows) within the left ventricular wall

Fig. 1.6 Left ventriculography (RAO projection) of the first published patient with isolated left ventricular noncompaction. Demonstration of the huge and deep spaces within the left ventricular wall after contrast agent injection into the left ventricular cavity, illustrating their connections (arrows)

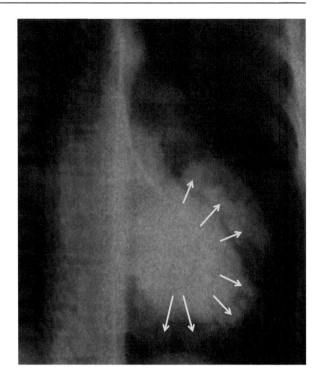

Symptoms and Diagnosis of NCCM

Since the symptoms in case of non-isolated NCCM are characterized by a broad spectrum of clinical presentation due to the accompanying congenital heart disease, patients with isolated NCCM usually show up with different symptoms. As already observed in the first case, the clinical entity in an adult patient sometimes includes only unspecific symptoms such as palpitations, but also complaints of heart failure symptoms, and supraventricular or ventricular arrhythmias as well as ECG abnormalities like complete bundle branch block and AV-block. In some cases thromboembolism may be present (Fig. 1.7).

Additionally, neuromuscular disorders and dysmorphism have been observed, especially in the pediatric population with NCCM [22].

Compared to adult patients, children with NCCM more often present with severe symptoms and a poor prognosis [50].

Detailed information on the clinical presentation in a larger cohort of adult and pediatric patients with NCCM is described in Chaps. 3, 4, 7, and 9.

The diagnostic method of choice in NCCM is echocardiography, which is widely available, not harmful and cost-effective. As our group reported earlier, the combined application of the "Swiss" and "Vienna" criteria can improve the echocardiographic diagnosis of NCCM ("German criteria") [46, 51–53].

Fig. 1.7 Autopsy specimen of a patient with left ventricular noncompaction, who died from sudden cardiac death. Thrombus formation (arrow), located in the trabeculated myocardium near the left ventricular apex

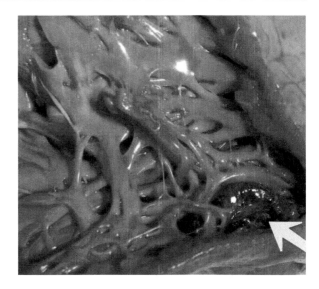

Fig. 1.8 Color coded echocardiography of a patient with left ventricular noncompaction. Left ventricle in the apical 4-chamber view. Blood flow from the left ventricular cavity into the intertrabecular spaces are clearly demonstrated (arrows)

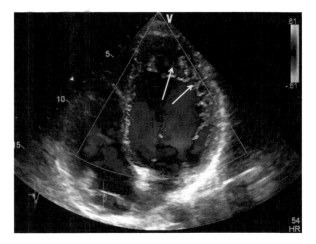

When needed, echocardiography may be supplemented by cardiac MRI or by other diagnostic tools (Figs. 1.8 and 1.9). But uniformly accepted diagnostic criteria are still missing (Fig. 1.2).

A detailed analysis of current diagnostic criteria of NCCM is described in Chap. 2.

Modern imaging techniques, especially echocardiography and cardiac MRI, with their high spatial resolution and delineation power allow the visualization of even fine trabeculations, quite often strictly localized to the ventricular apex. In our experience, this may be more frequently observed in top athletes, or other younger and healthy persons, depending on their ethnic origin. Therefore, it is of great

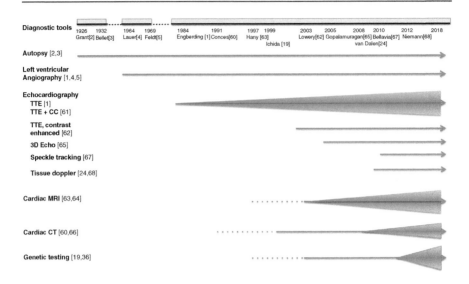

Fig. 1.9 Historical overview: important diagnostic modalities in left ventricular noncompaction. *TTE* transthoracic echocardiography, *CC* color coded

importance, to distinguish harmless phenotypes from pathologic myocardial remodeling and from NCCM. Interestingly, a recent study revealed that, independent from the extent of even excessive left ventricular trabeculation in asymptomatic patients, no deterioration of the left ventricular function during a 9.5 years follow-up could be observed [54]. As mentioned before, especially in this context, genetic testing may play a significant role in the future. Additionally, new data enhance the evidence, that the combination of genetic finding, clinical presentation and myocardial performance significantly determine the prognosis of the affected patients. This may offer a crucial improvement of the management of the disease [48, 49].

Detailed information on these problems are presented in Chaps. 8 and 9.

Conclusion and Future Perspective

Without a review of the historical background of a medical problem, the current concepts in diagnosis and management of a disease entity cannot be understood completely.

LVNC or NCCM are a rather new cardiac abnormality characterized by a typical pattern of apparently embryonic myocardial morphology. It can be detected by echocardiography as shown on the first case of isolated NCCM. Today, especially cardiac MRI represents an important additional diagnostic tool.

In the future, genetic testing may help in distinguishing a phenotype presenting with the typical trabecular myocardial pattern (LVNC) due to a physiologic or pathologic myocardial remodeling from the established noncompaction cardiomyopathy (NCCM), which is typically accompanied by left ventricular dysfunction,

ECG-abnormalities, symptoms of heart failure, supraventricular and/or ventricular arrhythmias and thrombembolism, or by a family history of NCCM.

Since ongoing research is still enhancing our knowledge and understanding of the normal embryonic development of the human heart, the insights in etiology, pathophysiology, genetic determination, clinical presentation and management of LVNC and NCCM will further increase [55]. A new study suggests, that combined data on the genetic findings, clinical presentation and myocardial performance improve the risk stratification of the disease [48, 49].

Future research to answer the open questions is urgently needed; the detailed perspectives will be addressed in Chap. 11.

Since the prevalence of the disease seems low, further data from multicenter prospective/retrospective, national/international studies or registries are required [47, 53].

References

1. Engberding R, Bender F. Identification of a rare congenital anomaly of the myocardium by two-dimensional echocardiography: persistence of isolated myocardial sinusoids. Am J Cardiol. 1984;53:1733–4.
2. Grant RT. An unusual anomaly of the coronary vessels in the malformed heart of a child. Heart. 1926;1:273–83.
3. Bellet S, Gouley BA. Congenital heart disease with multiple cardiac anomalies. Report of a case showing aortic atresia, fibrous scar in myocardium and embryonal sinusoidal remains. Am J Med Sci. 1932;183:458–65.
4. Lauer RM, Fink HP, Petry EL, Dunn MI, Diehl AM. Angiographic demonstration of intramyocardial sinusoids in pulmonary-valve atresia with intact ventricular septum and hypoplastic right ventricle. N Engl J Med. 1964;271:68–72.
5. Feldt RH, Rahimtoola SH, Davis GD, Swan HJ, Titus JL. Anomalous ventricular myocardial patterns in a child with complex congenital heart disease. Am J Cardiol. 1969;23:732–4.
6. Jenni R, Goebel N, Tartini R, Schneider J, Arbenz U, Oelz O. Persisting myocardial sinusoids of both ventricles as an isolated anomaly: echocardiographic, angiographic, and pathologic anatomical findings. Cardiovasc Intervent Radiol. 1986;9:127–31.
7. Chin TK, Perloff JK, Williams RG, Jue K, Mohrmann R. Isolated noncompaction of left ventricular myocardium. A study of eight cases. Circulation. 1990;82:507–13.
8. Dusek J, Ostádal B, Duskova M. Postnatal persistence of spongy myocardium with embryonic blood supply. Arch Pathol. 1975;99:312–7.
9. Harvey RP. Patterning the vertebrate heart. Nat Rev Genet. 2002;7:544–56.
10. Srivastava D, Olson EN. A genetic blueprint for cardiac development. Nature. 2000;407:221–6.
11. Eisenberg LM, Markwald RR. Cellular recruitment and the development of the myocardium. Dev Biol. 2004;274:225–32.
12. Agmon Y, Connolly HM, Olson LJ, Khandheria BK, Seward JB. Noncompaction of the ventricular myocardium. J Am Soc Echocardiogr. 1999;12:859–63.
13. Bernanke DH, Velkey JM. Development of the coronary blood supply: changing concepts and current ideas. Anat Rec. 2002;269:198–208.
14. Freedom RM, Yoo SJ, Perrin D, Taylor G, Petersen S, Anderson RH. The morphological spectrum of ventricular noncompaction. Cardiol Young. 2005;15:345–64.
15. Sedmera D, McQuinn T. Embryogenesis of the heart muscle. Heart Fail Clin. 2008;4:235–45.
16. Henderson DJ, Anderson RH. The development and structure of the ventricles in the human heart. Pediatr Cardiol. 2009;30:588–96.

17. Schleich JM, Abdulla T, Summers R, Houyel L. An overview of cardiac morphogenesis. Une anthologie du développement cardiaque normal. Arch Cardiovasc Dis. 2013;106:612–23.
18. Srivastava D. Making or breaking the heart: from lineage determination to morphogenesis. Cell. 2006;126:1037–48.
19. Ichida F, Hamamichi Y, Miyawaki T, Ono Y, Kamiya T, Akagi T, Hamada H, Hirose O, Isobe T, Yamada K, Kurotobi S, Mito H, Miyake T, Murakami Y, Nishi T, Shinohara M, Seguchi M, Tashiro S, Tomimatsu H. Clinical features of isolated noncompaction of the ventricular myocardium: long-term clinical course, hemodynamic properties, and genetic background. J Am Coll Cardiol. 1999;34:233–40.
20. Bennett CE, Freudenberger R. The current approach to diagnosis and management of left ventricular noncompaction cardiomyopathy: review of the literature. Cardiol Res Pract. 2016;2016:5172308.
21. Paterick TE, Umland MM, Jan MF, Ammar KA, Kramer C, Khandheria BK, Seward JB, Tajik AJ. Left ventricular noncompaction: a 25-year odyssey. J Am Soc Echocardiogr. 2012;25:363–75.
22. Finsterer J, Stöllberger C, Towbin JA. Left ventricular noncompaction cardiomyopathy: cardiac, neuromuscular, and genetic factors. Nat Rev Cardiol. 2017;14:224–37.
23. Engberding R, Stöllberger C, Gerecke BJ. Left ventricular noncompaction: affected wall regions in respect to LV function – data from the German Noncompaction Registry (ALKK). Circulation. 2012;126(Suppl. 21):A14830.
24. van Dalen BM, Caliskan K, Soliman OII, Nemes A, Vletter WB, ten Cate FJ, Geleijnse ML. Left ventricular solid body rotation in non-compaction cardiomyopathy: a potential new objective and quantitative functional diagnostic criterion? Eur J Heart Fail. 2008;10:1088–93.
25. Sanchez-Quintana D, Garcia-Martinez V, Climent V, Hurle JM. Morphological changes in the normal pattern of ventricular myoarchitecture in the developing human heart. Anat Rec. 1995;243:483–95.
26. Gittenberger-de Groot AC. Mannheimer lecture. The quintessence of the making of the heart. Cardiol Young. 2003;13:175–83.
27. Christoffels VM, Habets PE, Franco D, Campione M, de Jong F, Lamers WH, Bao ZZ, Palmer S, Biben C, Harvey RP, Moorman AF. Chamber formation and morphogenesis in the developing mammalian heart. Dev Biol. 2000;223:266–78.
28. Van Mierop LH, Kutsche LM. Development of the ventricular septum of the heart. Heart Vessel. 1985;1:114–9.
29. Jensen B, van der Wal AC, Moorman AFM, Christoffels VM. Excessive trabeculations in noncompaction do not have the embryonic identity. Int J Cardiol. 2017;227:325–30.
30. Sizarov A, Ya J, de Boer BA, Lamers WH, Christoffels VM, Moorman AF. Formation of the buildingplan of the human heart: morphogenesis, growth, and differentiation. Circulation. 2011;123:1125–35.
31. Sizarov A, Devalla HD, Anderson RH, Passier R, Christoffels VM, Moorman AF. Molecular analysis of the patterning of the conduction tissues in the developing human heart. Circ Arrhythm Electrophysiol. 2011;4:532–42.
32. Jensen B, Agger P, de Boer BA, Oostra RJ, Pedersen M, van der Wal AC, Nils Planken R, Moorman AF. The hypertrabeculated (noncompacted) left ventricle is different from the ventricle of embryos and ectothermic vertebrates. Biochim Biophys Acta. 2016;1863:1696–706.
33. Stöllberger C, Finsterer J. Trabeculation and left ventricular hypertrabeculation/noncompaction. J Am Soc Echocardiogr. 2004;17:1120–1.
34. Maron BJ, Towbin JA, Thiene G, Antzelevitch C, Corrado D, Arnett D, Moss AJ, Seidman CE, Young JB, American Heart Association; Council on Clinical Cardiology, Heart Failure and Transplantation Committee, Quality of Care and Outcomes Research and Functional Genomics and Translational Biology Interdisciplinary Working Groups, Council on Epidemiology and Prevention. Contemporary definitions and classifications of the cardiomyopathies: an American Heart Association scientific statement form the council on clinical cardiology, heart failure and transplantation committee: quality of care and outcomes research and functional genomics and translational biology interdisciplinary working groups; and the council on epidemiology and prevention. Circulation. 2006;113:1807–16.

35. Elliott P, Andersson B, Arbustini E, Bilinska Z, Cecchi F, Charron P, Dubourg O, Kühl U, Maisch B, McKenna WJ, Monserrat L, Pankuweit S, Rapezzi C, Seferovic P, Tavazzi L, Keren A. Classification of the cardiomyopathies: a position statement from the european society of cardiology working group on myocardial and pericardial diseases. Eur Heart J. 2008;29:270–6.
36. Klaassen S, Probst S, Oechslin E, Gerull B, Krings G, Schuler P, Greutmann M, Hürlimann D, Yegitbasi M, Pons L, Gramlich M, Drenckhahn JD, Heuser A, Berger F, Jenni R, Thierfelder L. Mutations in sarcomere protein genes in left ventricular noncompaction. Circulation. 2008;117:2893–901.
37. Stöllberger C, Finsterer J, Blazek G. Left ventricular hypertrabeculation/noncompaction and association with additional cardiac abnormalities and neuromuscular disorders. Am J Cardiol. 2002;90:899–902.
38. Finsterer J, Stöllberger C, Schubert B. Acquired left ventricular hypertrabeculation/ noncompaction in mitochondriopathy. Cardiology. 2004;102:228–30.
39. Finsterer J, Stöllberger C, Schubert B. Acquired left ventricular noncompaction as a cardiac manifestation of neuromuscular disorders. Scand Cardiovasc J. 2008;42:25–30.
40. D'Ascenzi F, Pelliccia A, Natali BM, Bonifazi M, Mondillo S. Exercise-induced left-ventricular hypertrabeculation in athlete's heart. Int J Cardiol. 2015;181:320–2.
41. Gati S, Papadakis M, Papamichael ND, Zaidi A, Sheikh N, Reed M, Sharma R, Thilaganathan B, Sharma S. Reversible de novo left ventricular trabeculations in pregnant women: implications for the diagnosis of left ventricular noncompaction in low-risk populations. Circulation. 2014;130:475–83.
42. Anderson RH, Jensen B, Mohun TJ, Petersen SE, Aung N, Zemrak F, Planken RN, MacIver DH. Key questions relating to left ventricular noncompaction cardiomyopathy: is the emperor still wearing any clothes? Can J Cardiol. 2017;33:747–57.
43. Oechslin E, Jenni R. Nosology of noncompaction cardiomyopathy: the emperor still wears clothes! Can J Cardiol. 2017;33:701–4.
44. Arbustini E, Favalli V, Narula N, Serio A, Grasso M. Left ventricular noncompaction: a distinct genetic cardiomyopathy? J Am Coll Cardiol. 2016;68:949–66.
45. Oechslin E, Jenni R. Left ventricular non-compaction revisited: a distinct phenotype with genetic heterogeneity? Eur Heart J. 2011;32:1446–156.
46. Stöllberger C, Gerecke B, Finsterer J, Engberding R. Refinement of echocardiographic criteria for left ventricular noncompaction. Int J Cardiol. 2013;165:463–7.
47. Weir-McCall JR, Yeap PM, Papagiorcopulo C, Fitzgerald K, Gandy SJ, Lambert M, Belch JJF, Cavin I, Littleford R, Macfarlane JA, Matthew SZ, Nicholas RS, Struthers AD, Sullivan F, Waugh SA, White RD, Houston JG. Left ventricular noncompaction anatomical phenotype or distinct cardiomyopathy? J Am Coll Cardiol. 2016;68:2157–65.
48. Oechslin E, Jenni J. Left ventricular noncompaction from physiologic remodeling to noncompaction cardiomyopathy. J Am Coll Cardiol. 2018;71:723–6.
49. van Waning JI, Caliskan K, Hoedemaekers YM, van Spaendonck-Zwarts KY, Baas AF, Boekholdt SM, van Melle JP, Teske AJ, Asselbergs FW, Backx APCM, du Marchie Sarvaas GJ, Dalinghaus M, Breur JMPJ, Linschoten MPM, Verlooij LA, Kardys I, Dooijes D, Lekanne Deprez RH, IJpma AS, van den Berg MP, Hofstra RMW, van Slegtenhorst MA, Jongbloed JDH, Majoor-Krakauer D. Genetics, clinical features, and long-term outcome of noncompaction cardiomyopathy. J Am Coll Cardiol. 2018;71:711–22.
50. Jefferies JL, Wilkinson JD, Sleeper LA, Colan SD, Lu M, Pahl E, Kantor PF, Everitt MD, Webber SA, Kaufman BD, Lamour JM, Canter CE, Hsu DT, Addonizio LJ, Lipshultz SE, Towbin JA, Pediatric Cardiomyopathy Registry Investigators. Cardiomyopathy phenotypes and outcomes for children with left ventricular myocardial noncompaction: results from the pediatric cardiomyopathy registry. J Card Fail. 2015;21:877–84.
51. Engberding R, Yelbuz TM, Breithardt G. Isolated noncompaction of the left ventricular myocardium - a review of the literature two decades after the initial case description. Clin Res Cardiol. 2007;96:481–8.
52. Stöllberger C, Gerecke B, Engberding R, Grabner B, Wandaller C, Finsterer J, Gietzelt M, Balzereit A. Interobserver agreement of the echocardiographic diagnosis of LV hypertrabeculation/noncompaction. JACC Cardiovasc Imaging. 2015;8:1252–7.

53. Engberding R, Stöllberger C, Ong P, Yelbuz TM, Gerecke BJ, Breithardt G. Isolated noncompaction cardiomyopathy. Dtsch Arztebl Int. 2010;107:206–13.
54. Zemrak F, Ahlman MA, Captur G, Mohiddin SA, Kawel-Boehm N, Prince MR, Moon JC, Hundley WG, Lima JAC, Bluemke DA, Petersen SE. The relationship of left ventricular trabeculation to ventricular function and structure over a 9.5-year follow-up. J Am Coll Cardiol. 2014;64(19):1971–80.
55. Towbin JA, Jefferies JL. Cardiomyopathies due to left ventricular noncompaction, mitochondrial and storage diseases, and inborn errors of metabolism. Circ Res. 2017;121(7):838–54.
56. Petersen SE, Selvanayagam JB, Wiesmann F, Robson MD, Francis JM, Anderson RH, Watkins H, Neubauer S. Left ventricular non-compaction. J Am Coll Cardiol. 2005;46(1):101–5.
57. Belanger AR, Miller MA, Donthireddi UR, Najovits AJ, Goldman ME. New classification scheme of left ventricular noncompaction and correlation with ventricular performance. Am J Cardiol. 2008;102(1):92–6.
58. Jacquier A, Thuny F, Jop B, Giorgi R, Cohen F, Gaubert JY, Vidal V, Bartoli JM, Habib G, Moulin G. Measurement of trabeculated left ventricular mass using cardiac magnetic resonance imaging in the diagnosis of left ventricular non-compaction. Eur Heart J. 2010;31(9):1098–104.
59. Gebhard C, Stähli BE, Greutmann M, Biaggi P, Jenni R, Tanner FC. Reduced left ventricular compacta thickness: a novel echocardiographic criterion for non-compaction cardiomyopathy. J Am Soc Echocardiogr. 2012;25(10):1050–7.
60. Conces DJ, Ryan T, Tarver RD. Noncompaction of ventricular myocardium: CT appearance. Am J Roentgenol. 1991;156(4):717–8.
61. Jenni R. Echocardiographic and pathoanatomical characteristics of isolated left ventricular non-compaction: a step towards classification as a distinct cardiomyopathy. Heart. 2001;86(6):666–71.
62. Lowery MH, Martel JA, Zambrano JP, Ferreira A, Eco L, Gallagher A. Noncompaction of the ventricular myocardium: the use of contrast-enhanced echocardiography in diagnosis. J Am Soc Echocardiogr. 2003;16(1):94–6.
63. Hany TF, Jenni R, Debatin JF. MR appearance of isolated noncompaction of the left ventricle. J Magn Reson Imaging. 1997;7(2):437–8.
64. Weiss F, Habermann CR, Lilje C, Razek W, Sievers J, Weil J, Adam G. MRI in the diagnosis of non-compacted ventricular myocardium (NCVM) compared to echocardiography. Rofo. 2003;175:1214–9.
65. Gopalamurugan AB. Left ventricular non-compaction diagnosed by real time three dimensional echocardiography. Heart. 2005;91(10):1274.
66. Mohrs OK, Magedanz A, Schlosser T. Noncompaction of the left ventricular myocardium detected by 64-slice multidetector computed tomography. Clin Cardiol. 2007;30(1):48.
67. Bellavia D, Michelena HI, Martinez M, Pellikka PA, Bruce CJ, Connolly HM, Villarraga HR, Veress G, Oh JK, Miller FA. Speckle myocardial imaging modalities for early detection of myocardial impairment in isolated left ventricular non-compaction. Heart. 2010;96(6):440–7.
68. Niemann M, Liu D, Hu K, Cikes M, Beer M, Herrmann S, Gaudron PD, Hillenbrand H, Voelker W, Ertl G, Weidemann F. Echocardiographic quantification of regional deformation helps to distinguish isolated left ventricular non-compaction from dilated cardiomyopathy. Eur J Heart Fail. 2012;14(2):155–61.

Multimodality Imaging, Diagnostic Challenges and Proposed Diagnostic Algorithm for Noncompaction Cardiomyopathy

2

Osama I. Soliman, Jackie McGhie, Folkert J. ten Cate, Bernard P. Paelinck, and Kadir Caliskan

Introduction

Noncompaction of the left ventricle (LVNC) or noncompaction cardiomyopathy (NCCM), is a relatively new clinical-morpho-pathologic entity, first described by Engberding and Bender in 1984 [1]. It is characterized by a prominent trabecular meshwork and deep intertrabecular recesses communicating with the LV cavity. NCCM entity has been firstly recognized ante mortem thanks to the upcoming echocardiography. Knowledge of the disease has been accumulated over the past 35 years due to the emergence of new technical advances in several imaging modalities, increased awareness among the clinicians as well as improved genetic testing. Two forms of the disease should be recognized, an isolated form of the disease and a NCCM associated with other cardiac anomalies. To date, echocardiography remains the predominant diagnostic tool. The aim of this chapter is to discuss the advantages and limitations in the use of echocardiography for diagnosis of NCCM and outline some perspectives into overcoming these challenges. Furthermore, the incremental value of other imaging modalities will be presented. This chapter will provide the reader with a state-of-the-art and future aspirations in diagnostic aspects of NCCM. In addition, the potential to develop newer criteria for diagnosis of NCCM and future research opportunities will be discussed.

O. I. Soliman (✉)
Erasmus MC University Medical Center, The Thoraxcenter, Rotterdam, The Netherlands

J. McGhie
Thoraxcenter, Department of Cardiology, Erasmus MC University Medical Center, Rotterdam, The Netherlands

The Euro Heart Foundation, Brussels, Belgium

B. P. Paelinck
Department of Cardiology, University of Antwerp, Antwerp, Belgium

K. Caliskan · F. J. ten Cate
Erasmus MC University Medical Center, Department of Cardiology, Rotterdam, The Netherlands

© Springer Nature Switzerland AG 2019
K. Caliskan et al. (eds.), *Noncompaction Cardiomyopathy*,
https://doi.org/10.1007/978-3-030-17720-1_2

Classifications of NCCM

There are two proposals for classification of NCCM; the 2006 American Heart Association (AHA) [2] and the 2008 European Society of Cardiology (ESC) classification of cardiomyopathies [3]. NCCM is considered a distinct primary genetic cardiomyopathy by the AHA [2]. In contrast, according to the ESC, it is not clear whether NCCM is a separate cardiomyopathy, or merely a congenital or an acquired morphological trait shared by many phenotypically distinct cardiomyopathies [3].

Diagnosis of NCCM

Appropriate clinical diagnosis is of uttermost importance in the clinical management of the individual patients, given the different therapeutic and prognostic strategies.

Furthermore, there are minimal requirements of potential diagnostic tools that are needed to establish diagnosis of NCCM.

To date a clear pathoanatomic definition of noncompaction cardiomyopathy is lacking due to paucity of data. However, a comprehensive cardiovascular examination (Table 2.1) is recommended to establish the diagnosis of NCCM.

History and Physical Examination

A standard cardiovascular work-up in the assessment of a patient with suspected NCCM includes a thorough personal and familial history and physical examination. It is important to take into consideration that athletes' heart may have a benign form of excess trabeculation. Neuromuscular examination is required particularly in children with suspected NCCM to rule out associated neuromuscular disorders and in patients with signs or symptoms of neuromuscular diseases.

Table 2.1 Key tools required for the establishment of an accurate NCCM diagnosis

- History and physical examination including
  - Family history of NCCM, heart failure, sudden cardiac death or myopathies
  - Ethnicity, race
  - Intensive sports/athleticity
  - Neuromuscular diseases
- ECG (arrhythmias and conduction abnormalities)
- Holter monitoring
- Exercise stress test
- Echocardiography (the primary modality of choice for screening and diagnosis)
- Cardiac MRI (increasing utility, second in line after echocardiography, accurate, assessment of underlying fibrosis)
- Cardiac CT (potential role, accurate, provides incremental information over coronary artery disease)
- Positron Emission Tomography (PET) (Perfusion)
- Angiography
  - Coronary angiography (excluding coronary arterial diseases, aberrant coronary arteries)
  - Left ventriculography (intra-trabecular recesses)
- Genetic testing (genotype-phenotype matching and prognosis)

Electrocardiographic Abnormalities

Nearly 90% of children and adults with NCCM have abnormal electrocardiographic (ECG) findings [4–9]. Unfortunately, none of the ECG abnormalities is specific to the disease but may be more related to the severity of the cardiomyopathy. However, the frequency of ECG abnormalities could differ with change in the disease severity and development of more severe LV dysfunction and heart failure.

A detailed analysis of current ECG findings of NCCM is described in Chap. 6.

Imaging

Currently, there are several imaging modalities that can help in the assessment of patients suspected with NCCM. In the following part, we will revise and discuss the currently used diagnostic modalities.

Conventional Echocardiographic Diagnostic Tools

Transthoracic echocardiography is the primary imaging modality. It can be used for screening, establishment of the diagnosis and monitoring of cardiac function [10, 11]. There are several echocardiographic modes that can be used in the assessment of suspected patients with NCCM (Table 2.2).

Diagnostic Criteria

Several echocardiographic and MRI derived criteria for the diagnosis of NCCM have been proposed (Table 2.5) [11–16]. There are 5 key morphologic features of NCCM that

Table 2.2 Key uses of different transthoracic echocardiographic modalities

Modality	Utility in NCCM
2D TTE	Initial screening, often provides the first clue or definitive diagnosis of NCCM in the majority of patients
M-mode	Best used for ventricular function, left ventricular mass assessment, less robust but has best image resolution
Doppler	The only modality, which provides hemodynamic and valvular regurgitation assessment. Thereafter, color Doppler confirmation of the deep intertrabecular recesses of the noncompacted myocardium
Bi-Plane	Provides an orthogonal display of the region of interest. i.e., LV, LA, MV annulus...etc.
SMPI[a]	Provides a comprehensive (360°) panorama of the entire ventricular walls as well as a more robust chamber and anatomic quantification
3D-TTE	Complete visualization of endocardial morphology as well as an accurate valvular and chamber quantification
Contrast Echocardiography	Provides proof of blood continuity between LV cavity and intertrabecular recesses, provides better visualization of LV cavity and wall motion assessment

[a]Simultaneous multiplane imaging

are described in part or all by published suggested criteria namely: (1) the presence of a two layered myocardial structure; (2) increased ratio of non-compacted (NC) to compacted (C) layer; (3) evidence of intertrabecular recesses communication with LV cavity; (4) absence (isolated) of or associated with other congenital or acquired heart disease and (5) preferential location and distribution of excess trabeculations.

Different research groups used either echocardiography or MRI based on their expertise. In addition, NCCM criteria differed being based on either measurement of NC to C thickness or NC to C area or NC to C mass. Those measurements are either performed on the short-axis (cross-sectional) or long-axis (sagital or coronal) views or both, at the systolic or diastolic phase or both. Despite all published criteria, more questions and uncertainties remain and NCCM or LVNC remains a difficult diagnostic entity.

Echocardiographic Criteria

We describe in this chapter the eight echocardiographic criteria widely used for diagnosis of NCCM.

- California criteria: Chin et al. referred (or named) in 1990 to the disease entity as isolated LV non-compaction (IVNC) since absence of associated congenital cardiac malformations was required for diagnosis [12]. The authors studied 8 patients including 3 patients at autopsy. Patients with the disease entity had excess trabeculations in LV apex and LV free wall with deep intertrabecular recesses communicates with LV cavity forming a 2-Layered myocardial structure. IVNC was defined by the presence of X/Y <0.5 at end-diastole in the parasternal short-axis view at the level of papillary muscle through and/or apical level, where: X = distance from the epicardial surface to the trabecular recess; Y = distance from the epicardial surface to the peak of trabeculation. This ratio could be translated to the NC to C ratio >2 adopted by most of the other NCCM criteria (Fig. 2.1).

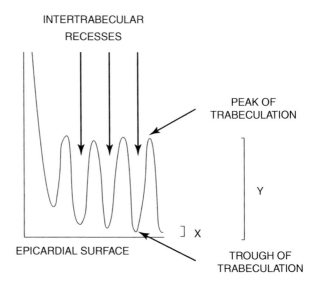

Fig. 2.1 California echocardiographic criteria. Chin et al. describes the method for determining X-to-Y ratio in 8 cases where X is the compacted myocardium defined as the distance from epicardium to the trough of the intertrabecular recesses. Y is the depth of the intertrabecular recess defined as the distance between peak and trough of intertrabecular recess that is equal to the depth of intertrabecular recesses. Reproduced with permission from Chin et al. [12]

- Zurich criteria: A decade later, Oechslin et al. [10] in year 2000 and Jenni et al. in year 2001 in analogy of Chin et al. [12] proposed new criteria to define IVNC based on anatomical validation of echocardiographic findings in 7 patients [10, 11] In absence of co-existing cardiac abnormalities, four findings were required to establish the diagnosis of IVNC: (1) Coexisting cardiac abnormalities were absent; (2) A two-layer structure, with a compacted thin epicardial band and a much thicker non-compacted endocardial layer of trabecular meshwork with deep endomyocardial spaces. A maximal end-systolic ratio of NC to C layers of >2 is diagnostic; (3) The predominant localization of the pathology was to mid-lateral (seven of seven patients), apical (six), and mid-inferior (seven) areas; (4) There was a color Doppler evidence of deep perfused intertrabecular recesses. These criteria are similar to Chin et al. criteria except in the end-systolic timing of measurements of excess trabeculations [11]. In addition, the authors referred to the IVNC as a congenital anomaly that is a distinct entity of cardiomyopathy (Fig. 2.2).
- Vienna Criteria: Stöllberger et al. [14] initially in year 2002 adopted the term LV hypertrabeculation (LVHT) to describe NCCM or LVNC. The authors focused on the number of LV trabeculations to diagnose LVHT. Two-dimensional and Doppler echocardiographic criteria for the diagnosis of LVHT were: (1) >3 trabeculations protruding from the left ventricular wall, apically to the papillary muscles, visible in 1 image plane; and (2) intertrabecular spaces perfused from the left ventricular cavity as visualized on colour Doppler imaging. Trabeculations are described as structures with the same echogenicity as the myocardium and moving synchronously with ventricular contractions. In a more recent analysis in 2013 by the same group [15], a refined criteria was used as follow: (1) >3 prominent trabeculous formations along the left ventricular endocardial border visible in end-diastole,

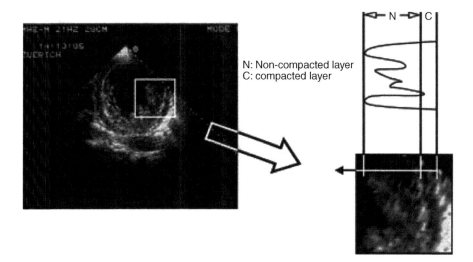

Fig. 2.2 Zurich echocardiographic criteria. Quantification of the extent of non-compaction at the site of maximal wall thickness, using the end-systolic ratio of non-compacted to compacted thickness. A two-layered structure is best seen in the short-axis parasternal view at end-systole. Reproduced with permission from Jenni et al. [11]

distinct from papillary muscles, false tendons or aberrant bands; (2) trabeculations move synchronously with the compacted myocardium, (3) trabeculations form the noncompacted part of a two-layered myocardial structure, best visible at end-systole; and (4) perfusion of the intertrabecular spaces from the left ventricular cavity is present at end-diastole on colour-Doppler echocardiography or contrast echocardiography. Interestingly, the authors reached a consensus that measurements of the thickness of the myocardial layers, and calculation of the NC/C ratio is not feasible due to a lack of uniformly accepted standards for measurements [17].

- New York Criteria: Belanger et al. [13] in year 2008 examined transthoracic echocardiograms from 380 patients for the presence or the absence of NCCM/LVNC. The authors had a very high 15.8% diagnosis of LVNC. Their methodology focused primarily on assessment of severity of LVNC by using the thickness and area of noncompacted regions. The presence, the ratio of the maximum linear length of noncompacted to compacted myocardium and the planimeter noncompacted area on apical 4-chamber view were used to classify subjects as healthy controls, or mild, moderate, and severe LVNC. As shown in the Table below, NC/C ratio of >0 but <1, 1 to <2 and 2 or more mark mild, moderate and severe NCCM, respectively. Likewise, NC area of >0 but <2.5 cm^2, 2.5 to <5 cm^2 and 5 cm^2 or more mark mild, moderate and severe NCCM, respectively (Table 2.3).

- German Criteria: Engberding et al. [18] in year 2010 proposed a combination of Zurich and Vienna criteria. The German Criteria require 4 Observations: (1) at least 4 prominent trabeculae and deep intertrabecular recesses; (2) blood flow between the LV cavity and the recesses is demonstrable with colour Doppler or through the use of contrast echocardiography; (3) 2-Layered myocardial structure, in which a NC to C ratio ≥2 in systole. Predominant location of trabeculation is in the apex, inferior, central, and lateral portions of the LV wall; and (4) No other cardiac abnormalities are present.

- Zurich modified Criteria: Gebhard et al. in year 2012 proposed an additional criterion to prevent overdiagnosis of NCCM. Maximal systolic compacted thickness <8 mm was found to be specific for NCCM and allowed the differentiation of NCCM from normal hearts as well as those with myocardial thickening due to aortic stenosis (Fig. 2.3) [19].

- Wisconsin Criteria. Pateriek et al. In year 2012 proposed a single criterion on 2D echocardiography based on end-diastole ratio of NC to compacted myocardium >2 on parasternal short-axis view for the diagnosis of NCCM. This could be measured as well on 2D-guided M-mode echocardiography (Figs. 2.4 and 2.5) [20].

- Rotterdam Criteria (Fig. 2.6)

Table 2.3 New York echocardiographic criteria

Classification of NCCM	NC/C ratio	LV NC area
None	0	0
Mild	>0 and <1	≥0 and <2.5 cm^2
Moderate	≥1 and <2	≥2.5 and <5 cm^2
Severe	>2	≥5 cm^2

Reproduced with permission from Belanger AR et al. New classification scheme of left ventricular noncompaction and correlation with ventricular performance. Am J Cardiol. 2008;102:92-96

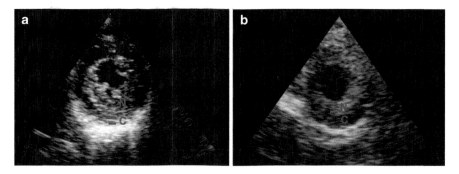

Fig. 2.3 Zurich modified echocardiographic criteria. Quantification of the noncompacted and compacted layers of the myocardium on the parasternal short axis view. Representative example of echocardiographic measurements in the parasternal short-axis view in a patient with NCCM (**a**) compared with one with aortic stenosis (**b**). *C* compacted myocardial layer, *N* noncompacted myocardial layer. Reproduced with permission from Gebhard et al. [19]

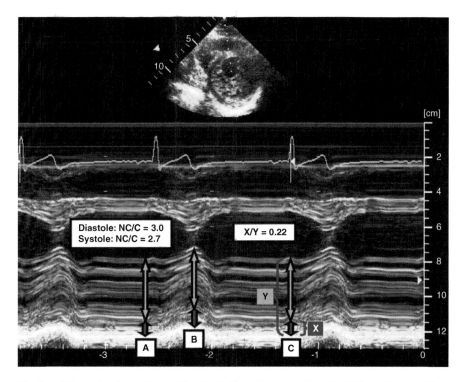

Fig. 2.4 Wisconsin echocardiographic criteria. Two-dimensionally guided M-mode images illustrating the different diagnostic criteria of NCCM. (**a**) Wiskonsin criteria: end-diastole: ratio of noncompacted (NC; green arrows) to compacted (C; blue arrows) myocardium = 3.0. Note that the NC myocardium has near identical thickness at end-systole and end-diastole, indicating an absence of radial thickening of NC myocardium. (**b**) Jenni criteria: end-systole: NC/C = 2.7. This end-systolic ratio of 2.7 is lower than the end-diastolic ratio because the C layer thickens radially at end-systole, while the NC myocardial thickness remains essentially unchanged, resulting in a reduced calculated ratio. (**c**) Chin criteria: end-diastole: compacted myocardium (X)/compacted plus noncompacted myocardium (Y) = 0.22. Reproduced with permission from Paterick et al. [20]

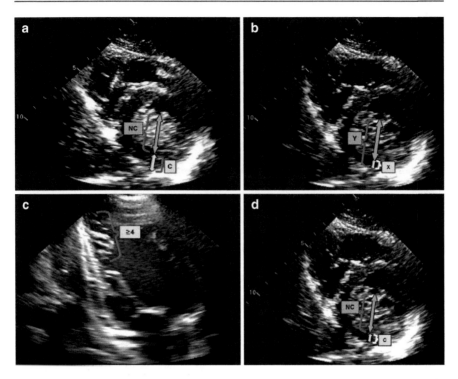

Fig. 2.5 Wisconsin echocardiographic criteria in comparison with other published criteria. Diagnostic criteria for LVNC. (**a**) Jenni (Zurich) criteria: NCCM is defined by a ratio of noncompacted (NC) to compacted (C) myocardium >2, measured at end-systole. (**b**) Chin (California) criteria: NCCM is defined by a ratio of the distance from the epicardial surface to the trough of the trabecular recesses (X) to the distance from the epicardial surface to the peak of the trabeculations (Y) < 0.5, measured at end-diastole. (**c**) Stollberger (Vienna) criteria: LVNC is defined by trabeculations (four or more) protruding from the LV wall, located apically to the papillary muscles and visible in one imaging plane. (**d**) Wisconsin criteria: LVNC is defined by an NC/C ratio >2, measured at end-diastole. Reproduced with permission from Paterick et al. [20]

Our echocardiographic approach includes both conventional trabeculation criteria and septal thickness in establishing the diagnosis. The full diagnostic algorithm is outlined in Table 2.4.

Limitations of Echocardiographic Criteria

Despite being, the most commonly used imaging modality in establishment of NCCM diagnosis echocardiography has some limitations. Dependence on acoustic window as well endocardial border definition are well known issues. Furthermore, pathoanatomic correlation of echocardiographic findings was performed in only three patients by Chin et al. [12], nine patients by Oeschslin et al. [10] and seven patients by Jenni et al. [11] However, ongoing technological advances in echocardiography have significantly improved image quality and resolution. Therefore, more refined and standardized echocardiographic criteria in a larger patient population are currently warranted.

a

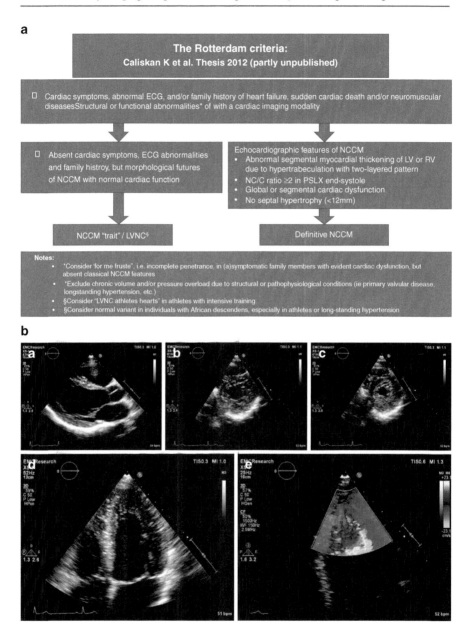

The Rotterdam criteria:
Caliskan K et al. Thesis 2012 (partly unpublished)

☐ Cardiac symptoms, abnormal ECG, and/or family history of heart failure, sudden cardiac death and/or neuromuscular diseasesStructural or functional abnormalities* of with a cardiac imaging modality

☐ Absent cardiac symptoms, ECG abnormalities and family histroy, but morphological futures of NCCM with normal cardiac function

Echocardiographic features of NCCM
- Abnormal segmental myocardial thickening of LV or RV due to hypertrabeculation with two-layered pattern
- NC/C ratio ≥2 in PSLX end-systole
- Global or segmental cardiac dysfunction
- No septal hypertrophy (<12mm)

NCCM "trait" / LVNC§

Definitive NCCM

Notes:
- *Consider 'for me fruste", i.e. incomplete penetrance, in (a)symptomatic family members with evident cardiac dysfunction, but absent classical NCCM features
- *Exclude chronic volume and/or pressure overload due to structural or pathophysiological conditions (ie primary valvular disease, longstanding hypertension, etc.)
- §Consider "LVNC athletes hearts" in athletes with intensive training
- §Consider normal variant in individuals with African descendens, especially in athletes or long-standing hypertension

b

Fig. 2.6 (**a**) The Rotterdam approach by Caliskan et al. Thesis 2012 (partly unpublished). (**b**) Patient with classic non-compaction cardiomyopathy. Echocardiographic assessment of NCCM showing a parasternal long axis view with normal septal thickness (**a**), a parasternal short-axis at the apical level showing trabeculations located anterior and posterior. (**b**, systole) and (**c**, diastole); the apical four-chamber view shows classic hypertrabeculations (**d**) and a color Doppler example of the flow pattern between the trabeculations (**e**)

Table 2.4 Summary of diagnostic criteria in NCCM

Echocardiography	
Chin et al. [12] (California criteria)	• Excess trabeculations in LV apex and free wall • Deep intertrabecular recesses communicates with LV cavity • 2-layered myocardial structure, NC to C ratio ≥2 • On the parasternal short axis view • Mid-LV and apical level • At end-diastole • No other congenital cardiac malformations
Öchslin et al. [10] and Jenni et al. [11] (Zurich criteria)	• Excess trabeculations in LV apex and free wall • Deep intertrabecular recesses communicates with LV cavity • 2-Layered myocardial structure, NC to C ratio >2 • On the parasternal short axis view • At end-systole • LV mid-level through apex mainly seen in apex, mid-lateral, mid-inferior • No other congenital or acquired heart disease
Stöllberger et al. [17] (Vienna refined criteria)	• >3 prominent trabeculous formations along the left ventricular endocardial border visible in end-diastole, distinct from (apically to) papillary muscles, false tendons or aberrant bands; • Trabeculations move synchronously with the compacted myocardium, visible in 1 image plane • Trabeculations form the noncompacted part of a two-layered myocardial structure, best visible at end-systole; and • Perfusion of the intertrabecular spaces from the ventricular cavity is present at end diastole on colour-Doppler echocardiography or contrast echocardiography • No measurements of the thickness of the myocardial layers, and calculation of the NC to C ratio should be performed due to a lack of uniformly accepted standards for measurements. • Apical four chamber view
Belanger et al. [13] (New York criteria)	• 2-Layered myocardial structure, NC to C ratio >2 • On the parasternal short axis view • At end-systole • LV apex, mid-lateral, mid-inferior • No other congenital or acquired heart disease
Engberding et al. [18] (German criteria) combination of Zurich and Vienna criteria	• There are at least 4 prominent trabecula and deep intertrabecular recesses • Blood flow between the cavum of the LV and the recesses is demonstrable with colour Doppler or through the use of contrast echocardiography • 2-layered myocardial structure, NC to C ratio ≥2 • In systole • Apex, inferior, central, and lateral portions of the LV wall • No other cardiac abnormalities are present
Gebhard et al. [19] (Zurich modified criteria)	• This group proposed an additional criterion to prevent overdiagnosis of NCCM • Maximal systolic compacted thickness <8 mm was found to be specific for NCCM and allows the differentiation of NCCM from normal hearts as well as those with myocardial thickening due to aortic stenosis [19]

Table 2.4 (continued)

Echocardiography	
Paterick et al. [20] (Wisconsin criteria)	• Proposed a single criterion on 2D echocardiography based on end-diastole ratio of NC to compacted myocardium >2 on parasternal short-axis view for the diagnosis of NCCM • This could be measured as well on 2D-guided M-mode echocardiography [20]

The Rotterdam criteria. Caliskan et al. Thesis 2012 (partly unpublished)	• Cardiac symptoms, signs, and/or ECG abnormalities in combination with morphological futures of NCCM, i.e.
	  – Abnormal myocardial LV and/or RV myocardial wall thickening in due to hypertrabeculation with a two-layered myocardium
	  – NC/C ratio >2 in PSLX end-systole
	  – Absent septal hypertrophy, i.e. <12 mm
	  – Absent chronic volume or pressure overload due to structural or pathophysiological conditions (i.e. longstanding hypertension, primary valvular disease, top athletes, etc.)
	  – Usually LV systolic dysfunction
	• If positive morphological futures of NCCM but normal cardiac function, and absent cardiac symptoms, family history, or ECG abnormalities: diagnose as benign NCCM "trait" or LVNC
	• Caution in patients with African descendant's and prominent hypertrabeculation, especially in combination with longstanding hypertension or intensive sports

MRI	
Petersen et al. [40] (United Kingdom)	• 2-Layered myocardial structure, maximal NC to C ratio >2.3 • True apex excluded • Long-axis or AP4CH • End-diastole
Jacquier et al. [21] (France)	• 2-layered myocardial structure, trabeculated NC mass >20% of the global LV mass • Short-axis and long-axis • End-diastole
MSCT	
Melendez-Ramirez et al. [44]	• 2-layered myocardial structure, maximal NC to C ratio >2.2 in ≥2 segments • True apex excluded • Short-axis • End-diastole

Comparative Studies of Echocardiographic Criteria

Kohli et al. [22] in year 2008 compared the California, Zurich and Vienna criteria in 199 adults with impaired left ventricular systolic function referred to a heart failure clinic. The authors found that 24% of subjects satisfied at least one of the three criteria for NCCM. In this study, only 7% of patients fulfilled all three criteria. Those findings reflect the limited utility of a single echocardiographic criterion as mentioned before. Therefore, combining key features of those criteria is important to avoid over or underdiagnosis. Furthermore, excess trabeculations should be regarded as a spectrum ranging from none to severe. Besides, overlap of trabeculations between NCCM and normal variants or other cardiomyopathies should be always considered.

Advanced Echocardiographic Diagnostic Tools

Technical advances in echocardiography allowed for the emergence of high resolution images as well as newer modalities such as contrast [23, 24], tissue Doppler imaging [25, 26], speckle tracking [27, 28], and three-dimensional echocardiography [29, 30]. These advanced modalities can improve our understanding of pathophysiologic aspects of NCCM as well as better and early diagnosis.

Contrast Echocardiography

Our group and others have shown that contrast-enhanced two- and three-dimensional echocardiography provide better endocardial border delineation in patients with NCCM (Fig. 2.7) [23, 24, 31, 32].

Tissue Doppler Imaging (TDI)

TDI allows quantification of radial and longitudinal, regional and global myocardial velocity and strain in patients with NCCM [25, 33]. Impairment of both systolic and diastolic TDI mitral annular velocities in patients with NCCM precedes impairment

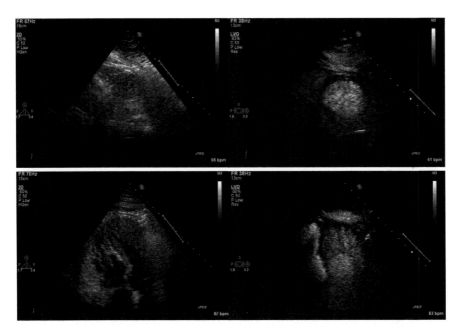

Fig. 2.7 Contrast echocardiography in a patient with non-compaction cardiomyopathy. Short-axis view of the left ventricle at the mid-ventricular level in a patient with non-compaction cardiomyopathy (top panel) and the apical 4-chamber view (lower panel): left panels: LV cavity is poorly visualized due to extensive trabeculations. Right panels: LV cavity is clearly seen after using contrast LV opacification. Intertrabecular recesses are filled with contrast

in LV ejection fraction. Furthermore, NCCM patients with an impaired early diastolic lateral mitral annular velocity have poor outcome [34].

Speckle Tracking Echocardiography

Bellavia et al. [27] found impaired LV rotation, twisting, and systolic strain in patients with NCCM despite normal LV ejection fraction and tissue Doppler measurements in some cases. LV rotation of the apical segments, LV torsion and torsion rate can accurately discriminate patients with NCCM from healthy controls. Furthermore, our group found that a functional pattern of rigid body rotation on speckle tracking echocardiography is associated with NCCM [28, 35]. This finding supports the congenital theory of NCCM origin. Rigid body rotation of LV reflects the abnormally developed myocardial layers resulting in absence of the normal helical fiber structure of the heart. In contrast, Pacileo et al. [36] showed prolonged but preserved LV systolic twist in 14 asymptomatic patients with NCCM similar to healthy controls. Impairment of LV strain, rotation and twist is related to NCCM severity which is supported by abnormal mitral annular geometry and impaired annular motion on three-dimensional echocardiography [29].

Magnetic Resonance Imaging

Currently, in patients with suspected NCCM, cardiac magnetic resonance imaging (MRI) is used as a second line tool if echocardiography is non-diagnostic. MRI provides excellent tissue-blood contrast resulting in better visualization of myocardial trabeculations. Furthermore, Cardiac MRI is the gold standard for assessment of LV function. In addition, MRI has the potential of tissue characterization including assessment of localized myocardial fibrosis using late gadolinium enhancement and diffuse myocardial fibrosis using T1-mapping (Fig. 2.8) [37–39].

MRI Criteria for NCCM

Authors used different criteria for the diagnosis of NCCM.

Petersen et al. in year 2005 proposed an end-diastolic ratio of compacted to non-compacted myocardium >2.3 in long-axis views for the diagnosis of NCCM [40].

Jacquier et al. in year 2010 proposed an end-diastolic ratio of >20% of LV trabecular mass compared to global LV mass to establish diagnosis of NCCM on MRI [21]. The authors used both long and short axis views to calculate trabeculation mass. To calculate global LV mass epicardial and endocardial contours were traced taking into account papillary muscles and trabeculations. To calculate LV compacted mass, LV trabeculations were excluded from tracing.

Limitations of MRI Criteria

Proposed MRI criteria were derived from small, selected populations. Another limitation of the MRI criteria is related to the slice selection and partial volume effects of single view MRI slices, which might lead to over/underestimation of the size and/or mass of trabeculations [21]. A recent finding of mid-myocardial fibrosis on MRI images in patients with NCCM, unrelated to noncompacted regions could open new areas of research towards better understanding of the disease [41].

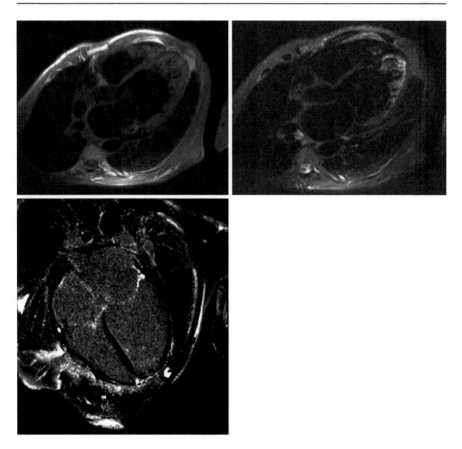

Fig. 2.8 MRI in a patient with NCCM. MRI in a patient with NCCM using T1 spin echo (top), T2 spin echo (middle) and late gadolinium enhancement (bottom)

Recently, Dawson et al. used cardiac MRI to separate normal LV trabeculation from pathological noncompaction in 120 volunteers. All had a visible trabeculated layer in 1 or more segments. Age- and sex-related morphometric differences were demonstrated in the apparent trabeculated and compacted layer thickness. Systolic thinning of the trabeculated layer was seen contrasting with compacted myocardial wall thickening [42].

Weir-McCall et al. [43] illustrated the use of four MRI criteria for diagnosis of NCCM in a large group of participants (n = 1480) with no history of cardiovascular disease. LVNC ratios were measured on the horizontal and vertical long axis cine sequences. All individuals with a noncompaction ratio of >2 underwent short axis systolic and diastolic LVNC ratio measurements, and quantification of noncompacted and compacted myocardial mass ratios (Fig. 2.7). Those who met all 4 criteria were considered to have NCCM. The study findings were interesting, where 14.8% met ≥1 diagnostic criterion for NCCM, 7.9% met 2 criteria, 4.3% met 3 criteria, and 1.3% met all 4 diagnostic criteria. Long axis noncompaction ratios were the least specific, with current diagnostic criteria positive in 14.8%, whereas the noncompacted to compacted myocardial mass ratio was the most specific, only being met in 4.4%. The authors concluded that those criteria have poor specificity for NCCM, or that LVNC is an anatomical phenotype rather than a distinct cardiomyopathy (Fig. 2.9).

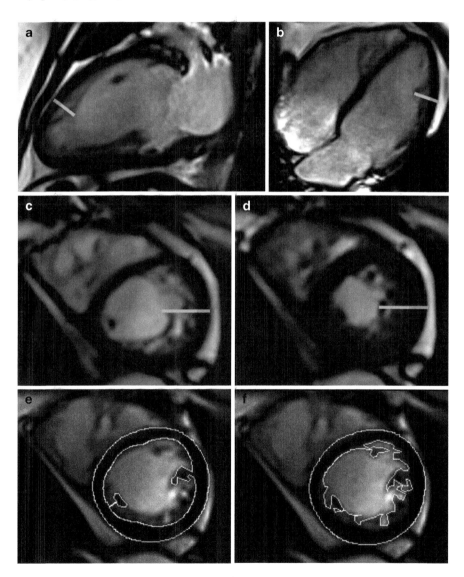

Fig. 2.9 Limitations of MRI criteria for diagnosis of NCCM. (**a, b**) Images demonstrate long axis noncompaction ratio measurement (orange line = compacted myocardium, blue line = noncompacted myocardium) with a maximum long axis noncompaction ratio of 3.4 obtained in the anterior apical wall. (**c, d**) Images show short axis noncompaction measurements are demonstrated at diastole (**c**) where the maximum noncompaction ratio = 3.6 and systole (**d**) where the maximum noncompaction ratio = 2.2. (**e, f**) Images delineate compacted and total myocardial mass contours giving a noncompacted mass of 24% of the total mass. Reproduced from the Weir-McCall et al. [43]

Cardiac Computed Tomography

There are scarce data on the use of computed tomography (CT) in the diagnosis of NCCM patients. Melendez-Ramirez et al. analyzed ECG-gated coronary CT angiography from 10 consecutive patients with NCCM diagnosed by echocardiography and/or MRI. The NC/C ratio in end diastole in each of the standard AHA 17 segments (excluding the apex) was calculated.

To determine the cut-off that would distinguish NCCM from other entities CT findings were compared with 9 healthy subjects, 14 patients with hypertrophic cardiomyopathy, and 17 patients with dilated cardiomyopathy. Based on these data, considering involvement of more than 1 segment, the NC/C ratio of 2.2 of ≥2 segments allowed the distinction of all patients with NCCM from other cardiomyopathies and from healthy subjects (Table 2.5) [44].

Table 2.5 Proposed diagnostic algorithm ("the Rotterdam Criteria") for suspected patients with NCCM using comprehensive cardiovascular and physical examination, echocardiography, and MRI in selected patients

• Step 1. Assess the clinical presentation
– Asymptomatic (by chance: e.g. abnormal ECG, chest X-ray, etc.)/familial screening
– Atypical chest pain
– Palpitations: no arrhythmias, frequent PVC's, or nonsustained SVT's/VT's
– Supraventricular arrhythmias e.g. atrial fibrillation, atrial flutter)
– Ventricular arrhythmias: sustained VT's (with or without syncope), VF (aborted sudden cardiac death)
– Sudden cardiac death
– Thrombo-embolic event
– Heart failure
• Step 1. Assess trabeculations as a continuum
– Normal (NC/C ratio in end-systole <1.0)
– Excess (NC/C ratio between 1.0 and 1.9
– Abnormal (NC/C ratio ≥2.0
• Step 2. Assess the extent and localization of the noncompacted (NC) segments
– Left, right, or biventricular involvement
– Maximal myocardial thickness (noncompacted + compacted)
– Maximal noncompacted/compacted (NC/C) ratio
– Involvement of noncompacted segments: use the 17-segments model
• Step 3. Assess functional, genetic and/or associated anomalies
– With or without structural heart malformations
– With or without LV dysfunction
– With or without RV involvement
– With or without RV dysfunction
– Genetic and familial association
– Arrhythmogenic and/or thromboembolic complications
• Step 4. Assign an LVNC/NCCM subtype (with or without a familial/genetic pattern)
– Benign LVNC
– Secondary LVNC (e.g. due to chronic volume or pressure overload)
– Asymptomatic NCCM
– NCCM with HFrEF (LVEF <40%)
– Arrhythmogenic NCCM (including VT/VF/aborted SCD)
– Predominant right ventricular NCCM (e.g. Phospholamban mutation)
– Biventricular NCCM
– Hypertrophic phenotype (mixed NCCM/HCM, especially with sarcomere gene mutations)
– Dilated phenotype (mild/moderate: classical NCCM)
– Restrictive phenotype (mixed RCM/NCCM)
– Associated with congenital heart disease
– Associated with neuromuscular diseases

Diagnostic Uncertainties

After three decades of research, the diagnosis of NCCM still represents a major dilemma [45]. The first dilemma is to distinguish normal variant(s) from pathologic trabeculations. It is important to recognize that the criss-crossing meshwork of thin muscle bundles at the LV apical segments are normal structures. Boyd et al. described that, any prominent trabeculation could be seen in up to 70%, while two or more prominent trabeculations are present in 36% of normal hearts [46]. False tendons are another normal variant, which are seen in 0.5% of normal hearts extending between the septum and the papillary muscles [47]. Furthermore, multiple bellies of the papillary muscle or additional papillary muscles may be present and should not be mistaken for pathologic trabeculations.

Next dilemma is to distinguish NCCM from other forms of cardiomyopathies. As mentioned before, NCCM exists as a disease spectrum ranging from mild to severe in both trabeculations severity as well as LV functional impairment. A hypertrabeculation pattern resembling NCCM was seen in 43% and 28% of patients with dilated cardiomyopathy and ischemic heart disease, respectively [48]. Furthermore, one or more of the echocardiographic criteria for NCCM were seen in 24% of patients of patients with systolic heart failure and in 8% of healthy subjects [22]. Likewise, a high incidence of prominent trabeculations is known in endurance athletes, patients with valvular heart disease, and blacks [22, 49].

The third dilemma is the mixed phenotype. Some patients with NCCM demonstrate a genetic and phenotypic overlap with HCM. Those patients might have both hypertrophy as well as pathologic trabeculations, but also, resembling mixed phenotypes [50].

Another key practical aspect of NCCM diagnosis, is the poor reproducibility of proposed imaging criteria of NCCM. In a recent study, the agreement of counting the number of trabeculations and measuring the ratio of noncompacted to compacted regions was only 67% [51]. Furthermore, the reproducibility of quantification of LV mass and LV noncompacted mass in patients with NCCM has been reported to be very poor [52]. Perhaps, this could be due to the slice thickness of MRI images and the lower spatial resolution of MRI compared to echocardiography.

Epidemiological Uncertainties

The lack of clear definition and still limited awareness of the disease entity among physicians precludes clear knowledge of disease prevalence. The prevalence of NCCM among adults has been reported as 0.014–0.26% of adults referred to echocardiographic laboratory [10, 53].

Practical Aspects

Despite three decades of research, many aspects of NCCM from the very basic definition to prognosis are not well defined. There is lack of clear consensus in the AHA and ESC guidelines [2, 3], on what should be described as NCCM and what is the position of NCCM among other cardiomyopathies [54, 55]. Our group supports the concept that NCCM is predominantly a genetic cardiomyopathy with variable morphological, functional, and clinical presentation.

The Trabeculations Continuum

First, it should be noted that the morphologic picture of NCCM is a continuum of LV trabeculations that extends from normal subjects to very severe forms of NCCM. There is no proof that any of the morpho-anatomic definitions is correct or could be applied to a general population including different ethnic groups, both genders, and to children and adults. New imaging tools, and in particular the use of contrast echocardiography, may be helpful [23, 24, 29, 56, 57]. In addition, there is a high prevalence of physiologic variants of trabeculations in blacks.

Second, the prevalence of NCCM depends on the applied criteria. Differences are probably related to the lack of anatomical landmarks, reproducibility and disease severity. A good example is the fact that the papillary muscles may be easily mistaken for NCCM in the short-axis view. Likewise, the relative thickness of myocardium is dependent on which phase of the cardiac cycle is used to measure the NC to compacted layer. Furthermore, apical abnormal muscle bands could be easily misdiagnosed as pathologic trabeculations. These pitfalls can be simply avoided via use of atypical views to exclude normal variants.

Severity of Trabeculations and LVEF Measurements

Deep trabeculations may represent a diagnostic challenge in evaluation of LV volumes and ejection fraction because of the inherent problems of the technique and the difficulties of tracing the true endocardium because of the trabecular structures. However, this issue is no longer a limitation when using the most recent MRI automated tracing software. In such situations, the use of wall motion score index, tissue Doppler echocardiography and speckle tracking imaging may be an alternative to assess LV function. However, an index or cut-off value of global and regional LV function is yet to be developed. Finally, the altered orientation of myocardial fibres in patients with NCCM could be challenge in the assessment of deformation imaging such as speckle tracking echocardiography.

Severity of Trabeculations and Long-Term Outcome

Andreini et al. [58] investigated 113 patients with NCCM from 5 centers using MRI and followed patients for a median of 4 years. The study endpoint was a composite of thromboembolic events, heart failure hospitalizations, ventricular arrhythmias, and cardiac death. The authors found that severity of trabeculations on MRI in patients with NCCM, has less prognostic significance for the composite endpoint than known heart failure parameters such as LV dilation, systolic dysfunction, or fibrosis. Those without these features had a favorable prognosis. Likewise, Caliskan et al. from our group investigated the severity and location of trabeculations in relationship with LV dysfunction [59]. A total of 29 patients in sinus rhythm and NCCM were compared to 29 age and gender matched healthy controls. Segmental radial wall motion of all compacted and noncompacted segments was assessed with the standard visual wall motion score index and longitudinal systolic wall velocity with tissue Doppler imaging of the mitral annulus. Interestingly patients with NCCM with and without heart failure had similar total and maximal noncompaction scores. Furthermore, impaired LV function as measured by longitudinal LV wall velocity was not related to the extent or severity of noncompaction [59].

Systolic Versus Diastolic Phase for Measurements of Trabeculations

The compacted layer increases in thickness at end-systole compared to end-diastole due to the contractile reserve of these region. In contrast, the non-compacted layer does not change in thickness during the cardiac cycle, which affects the sensitivity and specificity of different diagnostic criteria [20]. Jenni et al. used the ratio NC/C > 2 at end-systole, yielding higher specificity and lower sensitivity compared with Chin et al., who used the equivalent of C/NC + C < 0.5, including the compacted myocardium in the numerator and denominator, increasing the sensitivity but lowering the specificity compared with Jenni et al.

Diagnostic Algorithm and Future Perspectives

More definite answers on the nomenclature, classification, pathophysiology, and outcome are needed to define the NCCM disease entity. A large and prospective study or registry that considers a great number of patients with NCCM is a crucial step to clarify current uncertainties. Alongside, pathoanatomic correlation of the imaging data should be established in larger series. Due to the genetic heterogeneity and lack of clear view on the genotype-phenotype relationship of NCCM, more genetic counselling, DNA diagnostics, and cardiological family screening should be encouraged.

Based on pathologic, clinical, and genetic analysis, we propose a new algorithm for the assessment of suspected patients with NCCM. A new classification should clearly be defining:

(1) physiological trabeculations,
(2) prominent non-pathological or secondary trabeculations,
(3) possible NCCM, and
(4) definite NCCM

Two forms of the disease should be recognized, and isolated form of the disease and a NCCM associated with other cardiac anomalies. Parameters should not only include the absence of other diseases (congenital, valvular) and the size and location of trabeculations, but also LV functional parameters (impaired LV function, rigid body rotation, and genetics).

Highlights

- Noncompaction cardiomyopathy is a primarily genetic disease with a wide spectrum of phenotypic expression and widely variable outcome.
- A clear pathoanatomic definition of noncompaction cardiomyopathy is lacking due to paucity of data.
- Echocardiography is the primary imaging modality for suspected patients with NCCM. It has contributed to the awareness and understanding of many aspects of the disease.
- MRI is a complementary imaging modality. Delayed gadolinium enhancement with MRI can identify myocardial fibrosis, which may have prognostic implications.
- Computed tomography is complementary imaging modality to echocardiography. It provides images with superb resolution quality. More importantly, it provides assessment of eventual coronary artery disease.
- Over three decades, plethora of suggested diagnostic criteria have been proposed. However, a consensus is essential for the standardization of the disease in terms of diagnosis, severity, treatment strategies and prognosis.
- Before a consensus statement can be a reality, a large international, multicenter study or registry is needed to clarify several aspects of noncompaction cardiomyopathy. In this study, morphological and functional multimodality imaging along with genetic testing and clinical follow-up should be included.
- For the time being, we propose a step-wise diagnostic algorithm, incorporating the current knowledge of the literature and our own clinical experience of more than a decade.

References

1. Engberding R, Bender F. Identification of a rare congenital anomaly of the myocardium by two-dimensional echocardiography: persistence of isolated myocardial sinusoids. Am J Cardiol. 1984;53:1733–4.
2. Maron BJ, Towbin JA, Thiene G, Antzelevitch C, Corrado D, Arnett D, Moss AJ, Seidman CE, Young JB. Contemporary definitions and classification of the cardiomyopathies: an American Heart Association Scientific Statement from the Council on Clinical Cardiology, Heart Failure and Transplantation Committee; Quality of Care and Outcomes Research and Functional Genomics and Translational Biology Interdisciplinary Working Groups; and Council on Epidemiology and Prevention. Circulation. 2006;113:1807–16.

3. Elliott P, Andersson B, Arbustini E, Bilinska Z, Cecchi F, Charron P, Dubourg O, Kuhl U, Maisch B, McKenna WJ, Monserrat L, Pankuweit S, Rapezzi C, Seferovic P, Tavazzi L, Keren A. Classification of the cardiomyopathies: a position statement from the European Society Of Cardiology Working Group on Myocardial and Pericardial Diseases. Eur Heart J. 2008;29:270–6.
4. Habib G, Charron P, Eicher JC, Giorgi R, Donal E, Laperche T, Boulmier D, Pascal C, Logeart D, Jondeau G, Cohen-Solal A. Isolated left ventricular non-compaction in adults: clinical and echocardiographic features in 105 patients. Results from a French registry. Eur J Heart Fail. 2011;13:177–85.
5. Stollberger C, Blazek G, Dobias C, Hanafin A, Wegner C, Finsterer J. Frequency of stroke and embolism in left ventricular hypertrabeculation/noncompaction. Am J Cardiol. 2011;108:1021–3.
6. Ergul Y, Nisli K, Varkal MA, Oner N, Dursun M, Dindar A, Aydogan U, Omeroglu RE. Electrocardiographic findings at initial diagnosis in children with isolated left ventricular noncompaction. Ann Noninvasive Electrocardiol. 2011;16:184–91.
7. Steffel J, Kobza R, Oechslin E, Jenni R, Duru F. Electrocardiographic characteristics at initial diagnosis in patients with isolated left ventricular noncompaction. Am J Cardiol. 2009;104:984–9.
8. Pignatelli RH, McMahon CJ, Dreyer WJ, Denfield SW, Price J, Belmont JW, Craigen WJ, Wu J, El Said H, Bezold LI, Clunie S, Fernbach S, Bowles NE, Towbin JA. Clinical characterization of left ventricular noncompaction in children: a relatively common form of cardiomyopathy. Circulation. 2003;108:2672–8.
9. Salerno JC, Chun TU, Rutledge JC. Sinus bradycardia, Wolff Parkinson White, and left ventricular noncompaction: an embryologic connection? Pediatr Cardiol. 2008;29:679–82.
10. Oechslin EN, Attenhofer Jost CH, Rojas JR, Kaufmann PA, Jenni R. Long-term follow-up of 34 adults with isolated left ventricular noncompaction: a distinct cardiomyopathy with poor prognosis. J Am Coll Cardiol. 2000;36:493–500.
11. Jenni R, Oechslin E, Schneider J, Attenhofer Jost C, Kaufmann PA. Echocardiographic and pathoanatomical characteristics of isolated left ventricular non-compaction: a step towards classification as a distinct cardiomyopathy. Heart. 2001;86:666–71.
12. Chin TK, Perloff JK, Williams RG, Jue K, Mohrmann R. Isolated noncompaction of left ventricular myocardium. A study of eight cases. Circulation. 1990;82:507–13.
13. Belanger AR, Miller MA, Donthireddi UR, Najovits AJ, Goldman ME. New classification scheme of left ventricular noncompaction and correlation with ventricular performance. Am J Cardiol. 2008;102:92–6.
14. Stollberger C, Finsterer J, Blazek G. Left ventricular hypertrabeculation/noncompaction and association with additional cardiac abnormalities and neuromuscular disorders. Am J Cardiol. 2002;90:899–902.
15. Stollberger C, Gerecke B, Finsterer J, Engberding R. Refinement of echocardiographic criteria for left ventricular noncompaction. Int J Cardiol. 2011;165(3):463–7.
16. Stollberger C, Winkler-Dworak M, Blazek G, Finsterer J. Prognosis of left ventricular hypertrabeculation/noncompaction is dependent on cardiac and neuromuscular comorbidity. Int J Cardiol. 2007;121:189–93.
17. Stollberger C, Gerecke B, Finsterer J, Engberding R. Refinement of echocardiographic criteria for left ventricular noncompaction. Int J Cardiol. 2013;165:463–7.
18. Engberding R, Stollberger C, Ong P, Yelbuz TM, Gerecke BJ, Breithardt G. Isolated noncompaction cardiomyopathy. Dtsch Arztebl Int. 2010;107:206–13.
19. Gebhard C, Stahli BE, Greutmann M, Biaggi P, Jenni R, Tanner FC. Reduced left ventricular compacta thickness: a novel echocardiographic criterion for non-compaction cardiomyopathy. J Am Soc Echocardiogr. 2012;25:1050–7.
20. Paterick TE, Umland MM, Jan MF, Ammar KA, Kramer C, Khandheria BK, Seward JB, Tajik AJ. Left ventricular noncompaction: a 25-year odyssey. J Am Soc Echocardiogr. 2012;25:363–75.

21. Jacquier A, Thuny F, Jop B, Giorgi R, Cohen F, Gaubert JY, Vidal V, Bartoli JM, Habib G, Moulin G. Measurement of trabeculated left ventricular mass using cardiac magnetic resonance imaging in the diagnosis of left ventricular non-compaction. Eur Heart J. 2010;31:1098–104.

22. Kohli SK, Pantazis AA, Shah JS, Adeyemi B, Jackson G, McKenna WJ, Sharma S, Elliott PM. Diagnosis of left-ventricular non-compaction in patients with left-ventricular systolic dysfunction: time for a reappraisal of diagnostic criteria? Eur Heart J. 2008;29:89–95.

23. Stollberger C, Finsterer J. Superiority of contrast echocardiography over conventional echocardiography in diagnosing left ventricular hypertrabeculation/noncompaction. Am J Cardiol. 2007;99:145–6.

24. de Laat LE, Galema TW, Krenning BJ, Roelandt JR. Diagnosis of non-compaction cardiomyopathy with contrast echocardiography. Int J Cardiol. 2004;94:127–8.

25. Nemes A, Caliskan K, Geleijnse ML, Soliman OI, Vletter WB, ten Cate FJ. Reduced regional systolic function is not confined to the noncompacted segments in noncompaction cardiomyopathy. Int J Cardiol. 2009;134:366–70.

26. Tufekcioglu O, Aras D, Yildiz A, Topaloglu S, Maden O. Myocardial contraction properties along the long and short axes of the left ventricle in isolated left ventricular non-compaction: pulsed tissue Doppler echocardiography. Eur J Echocardiogr. 2008;9:344–50.

27. Bellavia D, Michelena HI, Martinez M, Pellikka PA, Bruce CJ, Connolly HM, Villarraga HR, Veress G, Oh JK, Miller FA. Speckle myocardial imaging modalities for early detection of myocardial impairment in isolated left ventricular non-compaction. Heart. 2010;96:440–7.

28. van Dalen BM, Caliskan K, Soliman OI, Kauer F, van der Zwaan HB, Vletter WB, van Vark LC, Ten Cate FJ, Geleijnse ML. Diagnostic value of rigid body rotation in noncompaction cardiomyopathy. J Am Soc Echocardiogr. 2011;24:548–55.

29. Nemes A, Anwar AM, Caliskan K, Soliman OI, van Dalen BM, Geleijnse ML, ten Cate FJ. Non-compaction cardiomyopathy is associated with mitral annulus enlargement and functional impairment: a real-time three-dimensional echocardiographic study. J Heart Valve Dis. 2008;17:31–5.

30. Caselli S, Autore C, Serdoz A, Santini D, Musumeci MB, Pelliccia A, Agati L. Three-dimensional echocardiographic characterization of patients with left ventricular noncompaction. J Am Soc Echocardiogr. 2011;25(2):203–9.

31. Nemes A, Geleijnse ML, Krenning BJ, Soliman OI, Anwar AM, Vletter WB, Ten Cate FJ. Usefulness of ultrasound contrast agent to improve image quality during real-time three-dimensional stress echocardiography. Am J Cardiol. 2007;99:275–8.

32. Krenning BJ, Kirschbaum SW, Soliman OI, Nemes A, van Geuns RJ, Vletter WB, Veltman CE, Ten Cate FJ, Roelandt JR, Geleijnse ML. Comparison of contrast agent-enhanced versus non-contrast agent-enhanced real-time three-dimensional echocardiography for analysis of left ventricular systolic function. Am J Cardiol. 2007;100:1485–9.

33. van Dalen BM, Bosch JG, Kauer F, Soliman OI, Vletter WB, ten Cate FJ, Geleijnse ML. Assessment of mitral annular velocities by speckle tracking echocardiography versus tissue Doppler imaging: validation, feasibility, and reproducibility. J Am Soc Echocardiogr. 2009;22:1302–8.

34. McMahon CJ, Pignatelli RH, Nagueh SF, Lee VV, Vaughn W, Valdes SO, Kovalchin JP, Jefferies JL, Dreyer WJ, Denfield SW, Clunie S, Towbin JA, Eidem BW. Left ventricular non-compaction cardiomyopathy in children: characterisation of clinical status using tissue Doppler-derived indices of left ventricular diastolic relaxation. Heart. 2007;93:676–81.

35. van Dalen BM, Caliskan K, Soliman OI, Nemes A, Vletter WB, Ten Cate FJ, Geleijnse ML. Left ventricular solid body rotation in non-compaction cardiomyopathy: a potential new objective and quantitative functional diagnostic criterion? Eur J Heart Fail. 2008;10:1088–93.

36. Pacileo G, Baldini L, Limongelli G, Di Salvo G, Iacomino M, Capogrosso C, Rea A, D'Andrea A, Russo MG, Calabro R. Prolonged left ventricular twist in cardiomyopathies: a potential link between systolic and diastolic dysfunction. Eur J Echocardiogr. 2011;12:841–9.

37. Araujo-Filho JAB, Assuncao AN Jr, Tavares de Melo MD, Biere L, Lima CR, Dantas RN Jr, Nomura CH, Salemi VMC, Jerosch-Herold M, Parga JR. Myocardial T1 mapping and extra-

cellular volume quantification in patients with left ventricular non-compaction cardiomyopathy. Eur Heart J Cardiovasc Imaging. 2018;19:888–95.

38. Zhou H, Lin X, Fang L, Zhao X, Ding H, Chen W, Xu R, Bai X, Wang Y, Fang Q. Characterization of compacted myocardial abnormalities by cardiac magnetic resonance with native T1 mapping in left ventricular non-compaction patients- a comparison with late gadolinium enhancement. Circ J. 2016;80:1210–6.
39. Wan J, Zhao S, Cheng H, Lu M, Jiang S, Yin G, Gao X, Yang Y. Varied distributions of late gadolinium enhancement found among patients meeting cardiovascular magnetic resonance criteria for isolated left ventricular non-compaction. J Cardiovasc Magn Reson. 2013;15:20.
40. Petersen SE, Selvanayagam JB, Wiesmann F, Robson MD, Francis JM, Anderson RH, Watkins H, Neubauer S. Left ventricular non-compaction: insights from cardiovascular magnetic resonance imaging. J Am Coll Cardiol. 2005;46:101–5.
41. Nucifora G, Aquaro GD, Lombardi M. Cardiac magnetic resonance for early detection and risk stratification of patients with non-compaction cardiomyopathy: reply. Eur J Heart Fail. 2011;13:1154.
42. Dawson DK, Maceira AM, Raj VJ, Graham C, Pennell DJ, Kilner PJ. Regional thicknesses and thickening of compacted and trabeculated myocardial layers of the normal left ventricle studied by cardiovascular magnetic resonance. Circ Cardiovasc Imaging. 2011;4:139–46.
43. Weir-McCall JR, Yeap PM, Papagiorcopulo C, Fitzgerald K, Gandy SJ, Lambert M, Belch JJ, Cavin I, Littleford R, Macfarlane JA, Matthew SZ, Nicholas RS, Struthers AD, Sullivan F, Waugh SA, White RD, Houston JG. Left ventricular noncompaction: anatomical phenotype or distinct cardiomyopathy? J Am Coll Cardiol. 2016;68:2157–65.
44. Melendez-Ramirez G, Castillo-Castellon F, Espinola-Zavaleta N, Meave A, Kimura-Hayama ET. Left ventricular noncompaction: a proposal of new diagnostic criteria by multidetector computed tomography. J Cardiovasc Comput Tomogr. 2012;6:346–54.
45. Anderson RH, Jensen B, Mohun TJ, Petersen SE, Aung N, Zemrak F, Planken RN, MacIver DH. Key questions relating to left ventricular noncompaction cardiomyopathy: is the emperor still wearing any clothes? Can J Cardiol. 2017;33:747–57.
46. Boyd MT, Seward JB, Tajik AJ, Edwards WD. Frequency and location of prominent left ventricular trabeculations at autopsy in 474 normal human hearts: implications for evaluation of mural thrombi by two-dimensional echocardiography. J Am Coll Cardiol. 1987;9:323–6.
47. Loukas M, Louis RG Jr, Black B, Pham D, Fudalej M, Sharkees M. False tendons: an endoscopic cadaveric approach. Clin Anat. 2007;20:163–9.
48. Keren A, Billingham ME, Popp RL. Ventricular aberrant bands and hypertrophic trabeculations. A clinical pathological correlation. Am J Cardiovasc Pathol. 1988;1:369–78.
49. Bhattacharya IS, Dweck M, Gardner A, Jones M, Francis M. Isolated ventricular noncompaction syndrome in a nigerian male: case report and review of the literature. Cardiol Res Pract. 2010;2010:539538.
50. Towbin JA, Lorts A, Jefferies JL. Left ventricular non-compaction cardiomyopathy. Lancet. 2015;386:813–25.
51. Saleeb SF, Margossian R, Spencer CT, Alexander ME, Smoot LB, Dorfman AL, Bergersen L, Gauvreau K, Marx GR, Colan SD. Reproducibility of echocardiographic diagnosis of left ventricular noncompaction. J Am Soc Echocardiogr. 2011;25(2):194–202.
52. Fernandez-Golfin C, Pachon M, Corros C, Bustos A, Cabeza B, Ferreiros J, de Isla LP, Macaya C, Zamorano J. Left ventricular trabeculae: quantification in different cardiac diseases and impact on left ventricular morphological and functional parameters assessed with cardiac magnetic resonance. J Cardiovasc Med. 2009;10:827–33.
53. Sandhu R, Finkelhor RS, Gunawardena DR, Bahler RC. Prevalence and characteristics of left ventricular noncompaction in a community hospital cohort of patients with systolic dysfunction. Echocardiography. 2008;25:8–12.
54. Elliott P. The 2006 American Heart Association classification of cardiomyopathies is not the gold standard. Circ Heart Fail. 2008;1:77–9.
55. Maron BJ. The 2006 American Heart Association classification of cardiomyopathies is the gold standard. Circ Heart Fail. 2008;1:72–5.

56. Gianfagna P, Badano LP, Faganello G, Tosoratti E, Fioretti PM. Additive value of contrast echocardiography for the diagnosis of noncompaction of the left ventricular myocardium. Eur J Echocardiogr. 2006;7:67–70.
57. Nemes A, Caliskan K, Soliman OI, McGhie JS, Geleijnse ML, ten Cate FJ. Diagnosis of biventricular non-compaction cardiomyopathy by real-time three-dimensional echocardiography. Eur J Echocardiogr. 2009;10:356–7.
58. Andreini D, Pontone G, Bogaert J, Roghi A, Barison A, Schwitter J, Mushtaq S, Vovas G, Sormani P, Aquaro GD, Monney P, Segurini C, Guglielmo M, Conte E, Fusini L, Dello Russo A, Lombardi M, Gripari P, Baggiano A, Fiorentini C, Lombardi F, Bartorelli AL, Pepi M, Masci PG. Long-term prognostic value of cardiac magnetic resonance in left ventricle non-compaction: a prospective multicenter study. J Am Coll Cardiol. 2016;68:2166–81.
59. Caliskan K, Soliman OI, Nemes A, van Domburg RT, Simoons ML, Geleijnse ML. No relationship between left ventricular radial wall motion and longitudinal velocity and the extent and severity of noncompaction cardiomyopathy. Cardiovasc Ultrasound. 2012;10:9.

Neuromuscular Disorders and Noncompaction Cardiomyopathy

3

Josef Finsterer and Claudia Stöllberger

Introduction

Noncompaction cardiomyopathy (NCCM), also known as left ventricular hypertra-beculation (LVHT), has been repeatedly reported in patients with diseases of the skeletal muscle and rarely also in patients with diseases of the innervating neurons (neuromuscular disorders (NMDs)) [1]. The first patient with an NMD in whom LVHT was detected was reported in 1996 [2]. It was a 33 years old male with Becker muscular dystrophy (BMD) [2] in whom LVHT was accidentally detected when undergoing cardiologic diagnostic work-up for suspected heart failure [2]. During the following years, LVHT was additionally detected in a number of other NMDs (Table 3.1). Presence of an NMD in patients with LVHT has clinical implications. This chapter summarises and discusses previous and recent findings concerning patients with NMDs in whom LVHT was found and LVHT patients in whom an NMD was secondarily detected (Figs. 3.1 and 3.2).

History

After the first description of LVHT in a patient with BMD in 1996 [2], LVHT was consecutively described in a number of other NMDs. These include Barth syndrome [4], dystrobrevinopathy [6], mtDNA-related mitochondrial disorders (MIDs) [8],

Author contributed equally with all other contributors.Josef Finsterer and Claudia Stöllberger

J. Finsterer (✉)
Krankenanstalt Rudolfstiftung, Messerli Institute,
Vienna, Austria

C. Stöllberger
2nd Medical Department with Cardiology and Intensive Care Medicine, Krankenanstalt Rudolfstiftung, Vienna, Austria

© Springer Nature Switzerland AG 2019   41
K. Caliskan et al. (eds.), *Noncompaction Cardiomyopathy*,
https://doi.org/10.1007/978-3-030-17720-1_3

Table 3.1 NMDs in which LVHT has been described so far

NMD	Mutated gene	Reference
Becker muscular dystrophy (BMD)	*DMD*	[2, 3]
Barth syndrome	*G4.5/TAZ*	[4]
MIDs (biopsy, biochemistry positive)	uk	[5]
Dystrobrevinopathy	*DTNA*	[6, 7]
mtDNA-related MID (nonspecific)	mtDNA (*ND1, tRNA*)	[8]
Zaspopathy	*LDB3*	[7, 9–11]
Myotonic dystrophy 1	*DMPK*	[12–15]
mtDNA-related MID (LHON)	mtDNA (*ND1*)	[16, 17]
Laminopathy	*LMNA*	[18, 19]
Myoadenylat-deaminase deficiency	*AMPD1*	[20]
Duchenne muscular dystrophy (DMD)	*DMD*	[3, 21]
Hereditary neuropathy	*PMP22*	[22]
MYH7 myopathy	*MYH7*	[23, 24]
Myopathy with spherocytosis	uk	[25]
Myotonic dystrophy 2	*CNBP*	[26]
Oculopharyngodistal myopathy	uk	[27]
Glycogen storage disease IV	*Gbe1*	[28]
Fabry disease	*GLA*	[29, 30]
Duchenne carrier	*DMD*	[31]
Multiminicore disease	*RYR1*	[32]
Barth syndrome (carrier)	*G4.5/TAZ*	[33]
nDNA-related MID	*DNAJC19*	[34]
Congenital fiber type dysproportion	*MYH7B*	[35]
Glycogenosis IIb (Danon disease)	*LAMP2*	[36]
mtDNA-related MID (nonspecific)	mtDNA (*COX3*)	[37]
Non-specific muscular dystrophy	uk	[38]
Core myopathy	*TTN*	[39–42]
nDNA-related MID	*GARS*	[43]
nDNA-related MID	*SDHD*	[44, 45]
nDNA-related MID	*HADHB*	[46]
EBS with muscular dystrophy	*PLEC1*	[47]
nDNA-related MID	*MIPEP*	[48]
Walker-Warburg syndrome	*POMPT2*	[49]

NOP number of patients so far reported, *MID* mitochondrial disorder, *EBS* epidermiolysis bullosa simplex, *uk* unknown

zaspopathy [9], myotonic dystrophy 1 [12], laminopathy [18], myoadenylat-deaminase deficiency, *PMP22*-related hereditary neuropathy [22], *MYH7*-myopathy [50], myopathy with spherocytosis [25], myotonic dystrophy type-2 [26], oculopharyngodistal myopathy [27], glycogen storage disease-IV [28], Fabry disease [29], multiminicore disease [32], congenital fiber type dysproportion [35], Danon disease [36], nDNA-related MID [44, 46], epidermiolysis bullosa simplex with muscular dystrophy [47], metabolic myopathy due to *MIPEP* mutations [48], and Walker-Warburg syndrome due to *POMPT2* mutations (Table 3.1) [49]. NMDs in which LVHT occurs with a high prevalence are MIDs and Barth syndrome.

Fig. 3.1 Echocardiographic apical four-chamber view showing a dilated left ventricle with hypertrabeculation/noncompaction of the left ventricular apex and lateral wall

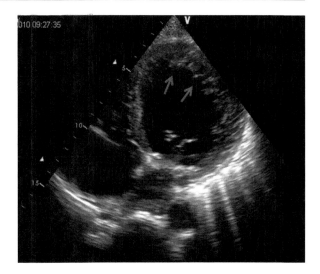

Fig. 3.2 Autopsy specimen showing hypertrabeculation of the posterior, lateral and apical segments in a patient with Duchene muscular dystrophy

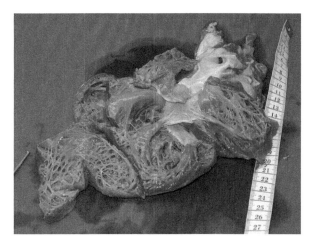

Mutated Genes Associated with LVHT and NMD

DMD

Mutations in the *DMD* gene may be asymptomatic or symptomatic. Clinical manifestations include Duchenne muscular dystrophy (DMD), one of the most prevalent muscular dystrophies in children, Becker muscular dystrophy (BMD), a milder form of DMD, and isolated dilated cardiomyopathy (DCM). Since the *DMD* gene is located on the X-chromosome, female carriers of a *DMD* mutation may also manifest clinically, depending on the random inactivation of the mutated/non-mutated chromosome. In DMD, BMD patients, and DMD-carriers, cardiac involvement is a common phenotypic feature. Most frequently, cardiac involvement includes conduction defects, arrhythmias, and DCM [51]. Only in single patients carrying a *DMD* mutation has LVHT been reported. The first patient carrying a *DMD* mutation and presenting with LVHT was a patient with BMD [2]. In 2005 the first patient with DMD and LVHT was reported [21]. In 2012 LVHT was reported for the first time in a female carrier of a *DMD* mutation [52]. Occurrence of LVHT in Duchenne carriers was confirmed in another case report [31]. In a study of 186 DMD/BMD patients, aged 4–64 years, from Japan, even 35 (19%) presented with LVHT [3]. Left ventricular function was worse among the 35 LVHT DMD/BMD patients compared to the 151 DMD/BMD patients without LVHT [3]. Over a follow-up of 46 months, on the average, left ventricular function deteriorated much quicker among the DMD/BMD patients with than without LVHT [3]. Additionally, the death rate during the follow-up period was much higher in the LVHT group (37% vs. 14.6%) [3]. In a study of 151 DMD patients from Italy, LVHT was detected in 15 patients (10%) [53]. In a study of 15 genetically confirmed DMD-carriers the rate of LVHT was 40% on cardiac MRI (cMRI) upon application of the Peterson criteria and 13% upon application of the Grothoff criteria [54]. One third of the females had systolic dysfunction and 60% had late gadolinium enhancement (LGE) [54].

G4.5/TAZ

The *G4.5/TAZ* gene encodes a protein, which is involved in the remodeling of cardiolipin. Tafazzin is highly expressed in the skeletal muscle and the myocardium [55]. Mutations in the *G4.5/TAZ* gene cause various different phenotypes, such as Barth syndrome, DCM, hypertrophic cardiomyopathy (HCM), endocardial fibroelastosis, and isolated LVHT. Barth syndrome is clinically characterised by the triad of DCM (or HCM, LVHT, or fibroelastosis), myopathy, and neutropenia [55]. Additional features include growth delay, exercise intolerance, cardiolipin abnormalities, and 3-methyl-glutaconic aciduria. The first report about LVHT in a patient with Barth syndrome dates back to 1997, when Bleyl et al. reported LVHT in 6 of 6 patients with Barth syndrome [4]. After this first description of LVHT in patients with Barth-syndrome [4], LVHT has been repeatedly reported in these patients and is now regarded as a hallmark of the disease [55]. Since Barth syndrome is an X-linked disorder, females transmit the disease and may be clinically unaffected or mildly affected. Also female carriers of the *G4.5/TAZ* mutation manifest in the heart. In 2012, LVHT was first described in a female carrier of Barth syndrome [33]. *G4.5/TAZ* mutations may show broad intra- and inter-familial phenotypic heterogeneity from severe Barth syndrome to asymptomatic LVHT with mild myopathy [56]. In rare cases, the hallmarks of the disease may be absent and patients may initially present only with growth retardation or mild myopathy [57]. In a study of 39 Japanese patients with LVHT, a pathologic variant was found in 16 genes [58]. In this study, *G4.5/TAZ* was the gene second most frequently mutated in LVHT patients (n = 6) after *MYH7* [58]. In a study of 36 pediatric patients with LVHT, two patients carried a *G4.5/TAZ* mutation [59]. In a Japanese study of 79 patients with LVHT, a TAZ mutation was detected in 2 of them [7]. When investigating a cohort of 34 patients with Barth syndrome, LVHT was diagnosed in 53% of them [60].

DTNA

The *DTNA* gene encodes for alpha-dystrobrevin, a component of the dystrophin-associated protein complex (DPC), which consists of dystrophin and several integral and peripheral membrane proteins, including dystroglycans, sarcoglycans, syntrophins, and alpha- and beta-dystrobrevin. *DTNA* mutations are associated with various congenital heart defects and LVHT. *DTNA* mutations were first described in association with LVHT by Ichida et al. in 2001 [6]. In a study of 70 Japanese patients with LVHT (20 familial and 59 sporadic cases), a *DTNA* mutation was found in only 1 family [7]. In a study of transgenic mice carrying an overexpressed *DTNA* mutation, deep trabeculations were found in addition to DCM with systolic dysfunction [61].

Mutated Genes Causing Mitochondrial Disorders (MIDs)

mtDNA Genes

mtDNA genes encode for subunits of respiratory chain complexes, for tRNAs, and for rRNAs. Of the 37 mtDNA genes, 4 have been reported in association with LVHT [1]. LVHT has been particularly reported in patients carrying mutations in *ND1* [62, 63]. In a Tunisian 16 years old female with hypothyroidism, work-up for cardiac compromise revealed tricuspid insufficiency, DCM, Ebsteins's anomaly, a superior caval vein draining into the coronary sinus, and LVHT [63]. The patient carried the homoplasmic variant m.3308T>C in the ND1 gene [63]. Studying mtDNA from 20 LVHT patients, a mtDNA mutation in the *ND1* gene was found in two of them [62]. In a study of 32 patients with a genetically confirmed MID (mitochondrial myopathy, n = 8, CPEO, n = 14, MELAS, n = 7, KSS, n = 2, MERRF, n = 1), 1 patient presented with LVHT due to a mutation in the *ND4* gene [64]. Isolated LVHT in a patient with Leber's hereditary optic neuropathy (LHON) has been first reported by Finsterer et al. in 2001 [16]. LHON in this patient was due to the variant m.3460G>A in the *ND1* gene [16]. Upon a family screening, LVHT was also detected in the brother of the index case, who also carried the *ND1* mutation m.3460G>A [17]. In a patient with mitochondrial myopathy due to the m.3243A>G mutation in *tRNA(Leu)* and nail-patella syndrome due to a *LMX1B* mutation, LVHT was detected [65]. Cardiac disease additionally included complete heart block, requiring pacemaker implantation [65]. Studies of the myocardium for mitochondrial changes from 6 LVHT patients revealed a *COX3* mutation in one of them [37].

nDNA Genes

GARS

Glycyl-tRNA synthetase (GARS) is an aminoacyl-tRNA synthetase (ARS) that links the amino acid glycine to its corresponding tRNA prior to protein translation and is one of three bifunctional ARS that are active within both the cytoplasm and mitochondria [43]. Dominant mutations in *GARS* manifest phenotypically as hereditary neuropathy or spinal muscular atrophy [43]. In a 12 years old female with exercise-induced myalgias persistent elevation of serum lactate and alanine, and periventricular leucencephalopathy, LVHT was detected upon screening for cardiac involvement [43]. The cause of the MID was a compound heterozygous mutation in the *GARS* gene [43].

HADHB

HADHB encodes for the beta-subunit of the mitochondrial trifunctional protein, an enzyme of the fatty acid beta-oxidation, which is built up of 4 alpha-subunits and 4 beta-subunits. Clinical manifestations of *HADHB* mutations are heterogeneous. The most severe phenotype is characterised by CMP, lactic acidosis, hypoketotic hypo-glycemia, and neonatal death [46]. LVHT has been reported only in one *HADHB* mutation carrier so far [46]. This patient was a fetus (third pregnancy of a Turkish lady) who's initial fetal echocardiography revealed biventricular hypertrophy, mild ventricular enlargement, but normal systolic and diastolic function. During the further pregnancy the fetus developed pleural effusions and edema due to systolic dysfunction [46]. After birth the child presented with severe lactic acidosis, being resistant to any therapy. Post-natal echocardiography revealed severely reduced systolic function and LVHT. The patient died shortly after birth without undergoing autopsy but genetic work-up of skin fibroblasts revealed a *HADHB* mutation [46]. The consanguineous parents did not exhibit phenotypic features of a MID and did not allow testing for the mutation [46].

MIPEP

The *MIPEP* gene encodes for the mitochondrial intermediate peptidase, an enzyme representing a critical component of the human mitochondrial protein import machinery, involved in the maturation of nuclear-encoded mitochondrial OXPHOS-related proteins (precursor processing) [66]. The mitochondrial intermediate peptidase is a mitochondrial pre-sequence protease, which processes about 70% of all mitochondrial pre-proteins that are encoded in the nucleus and imported post-translationally to mitochondria [48]. Mutations in the mitochondrial intermediate pre-sequence protease MIP/Oct1 have been recently found to cause a syndrome characterised by developmental delay, epilepsy, metabolic myopathy, severe hypotonia, cataracts, infantile death, and LVHT [48]. Muscle biopsy in three patients carrying *MIPEP* mutations from four unrelated families revealed moderate fiber size variation, type-1 fiber predominance, increased subsarcolemmal oxidative activity, increased number of mitochondria, pleomorphism of mitochondria on electron microscopy, marked increase in lipid droplets, increase in glycogen stores, membrane-bound glycogen deposits, and aggregation of mitochondria [48]. LVHT was found in two of the four patients so far reported [48]. In patient-1 LVHT was associated with WPW-syndrome and in patient-2 LVHT was associated with DCM [48]. Patient-1 was alive at age 4.5 years at the last follow up, having developed muscle hypertonia and dystonic movements. Patient-2 had died from intractable seizures at age 2 years [48].

SDHD

SDHD encodes for a subunit of complex-II of the respiratory chain. In a male neonate who had died 1 day after birth, post-mortem examination revealed HCM and LVHT [44]. Biochemical examination of the muscle revealed severe complex-II deficiency [44]. Genetic work-up revealed a recessive mutation in the *SDHD* gene [44].

DNAJC19

DNAJC19 encodes for a mitochondrial chaperone, located at the inner mitochondrial membrane. Mutations in this gene have been only rarely reported. The initial description is about a Hutterite family with DCM and ataxia [67]. LVHT in association with *DNAJC19* variants has been first described by Ojala et al. in 2012 in two Finnish brothers who additionally presented with DCM, microcytic anemia, male genital anomalies, and methyl-glutaconic aciduria [34].

Non-genetically Confirmed MID

Since the diagnosis of MIDs is challenging and not in each family a causative mutation can be detected, the diagnosis is often not genetically confirmed and based only on evidence, resulting from the phenotype, the lactate stress test, histochemical findings, and the biochemical results. Several cases of MIDs and LVHT without genetic confirmation have been reported. This is the case in a 31 years old female with mitochondrial myopathy in whom also LVHT was detected [68]. In a study of 113 pediatric patients with a MID, diagnosed upon the biochemical defect and in 11.5% upon a genetic defect, 13% (15 patients) had LVHT [69]. In a 6 weeks-old male with succinate-dehydrogenase deficiency, diagnosed upon muscle biopsy, echocardiography revealed not only DCM but also LVHT [67]. In a patient with complex-II deficiency LVHT has been reported in addition to DCM, failure to thrive, generalised hypotonia, and developmental delay [45]. The patient presented additionally with DCM, failure to thrive, hypotonia, and developmental delay [45]. In a study of 89 MID patients, diagnosed upon immunehistochemical and biochemical investigations, 33% had cardiac involvement [70]. In 3 of these patients, LVHT was detected [70]. In a female fetus, LVHT and AV-block 3 were diagnosed at 22 weeks' gestation [71]. Post-natally HCM and ventricular septal defects were additionally found and she received a pacemaker [71]. Muscle biopsy revealed a complex-I defect [71]. In a study of 220 patients with LVHT, a putative MID, diagnosed upon clinical, electromyographic, muscle bioptic findings, and lactate stress testing, was found in 19 patients [72]. The first MID patient in whom LVHT was detected was a 68 years male in whom muscle biopsy was indicative of a MID and in whom ventriculography, carried out during coronary angiography, revealed LVHT [5]. When studying 36 pediatric patients with LVHT, MID was diagnosed upon muscle biopsy findings in 5 [59]. Altogether, at least 62 MID patients with LVHT (mtDNA mutation: n = 8, nDNA mutation: n = 7, histochemical or biochemical evidence: n = 47) have been reported. Thus, MIDs seem to the NMD most frequently presenting with LVHT.

LDB3

LDB3 encodes for the Z-band alternatively spliced PDZ-motif protein (ZASP). ZASP is one of the major components of the Z-disc proteins in skeletal and cardiac muscle and plays an important role in stabilising the Z-disc through its PDZ-mediated interaction with alpha-actin-2 (ACTN2) and F-actin [10]. Mutations in *LDB3* manifest phenotypically as DCM, sudden cardiac death (SCD) myopathy, or LVHT [10]. LVHT has been first reported in three patients carrying a *LDB3* variant by Vatta et al. (Table 3.1) [9]. Additionally, LVHT was described in two patients with zaspopathy described by Xi et al. [10]. Xing et al. screened 79 patients with LVHT for mutations in *DTNA, SNTA1, FKBP1A*, and *LFB3*, and found a *LDB3* mutation in four of them [7].

DMPK

DMPK encodes for the dystrophia myotonia protein kinase, of which the specific function is unknown. However, there are indications that the enzyme has signalling and regulatory functions by interaction with other proteins, such as myosin phosphatase. The most well-known mutation in the *DMPK* gene is an intronic CTG-repeat expansion >49, clinically manifesting as myotonic dystrophy type-1 (MD1). Severity of MD1 correlates with the size of the CTG-expansion. Thus, the phenotype varies from an asymptomatic or only mildly manifesting condition to severe multisystem disease with early death shortly after birth (congenital myotonic dystrophy). The longer the CTG-expansion, the more likely becomes MD1 a multisystem disease, affecting all body tissues but particularly skeletal muscle, myocardium, endocrine organs, and the brain. Cardiac involvement in MD1 is frequent and mainly includes CMP and ventricular arrhythmias [13]. CMP may manifest as HCM, DCM, or as LVHT. LVHT has been first reported in 2004 by Stöllberger et al. [12]. Since then at least 25 other MD1 patients with LVHT have been described [12–15]. In a study of 40 MD1 patients, LVHT was detected in 35% of them (n = 14) [13].

LMNA

The *LMNA* gene encodes for lamin A/C, an intermediate filament protein associated with the inner nuclear membrane [73]. *LMNA* mutations result in abnormal cell signalling, which includes increased signalling by extracellular signal-regulated kinase-1 and kinase-2 and other mitogen-activated protein kinases, protein kinase B/mammalian target of rapamycin complex-1, and transforming growth factor-β [73]. Characteristic of *LMNA* mutations are that they show strong phenotypic heterogeneity manifesting as Emery-Dreifuss muscular dystrophy, limb girdle muscular dystrophy (LGMD), myofibrillar myopathy, DCM with conduction system disease, atrial fibrillation, or malignant ventricular arrhythmias, Dunnigan-type familial partial lipodystrophy, mandibulo-acral dysplasia, Hutchinson-Gilford progeria syndrome, restrictive dermopathy, or as autosomal recessive Charcot-Marie-Tooth disease type-2 [74]. LVHT in association with *LMNA* mutations has been first reported by Hermida-Prieto et al. in a single patient in 2004 [18]. Two Chinese patients carrying *LMNA* mutations and presenting with LVHT have been reported by Liu et al. in 2016 [19]. Unfortunately, it is unclear if these two patients also manifested in the skeletal muscles. LVHT in association with *LMNA* mutations has been also reported in 3 patients from the USA but again it remains unclear if these patients had an NMD or not [75]. In a study of 9 patients from 8 families carrying *LMNA* mutations, only 1 presented with LVHT. Phenotypic heterogeneity was broad among the 9 patients [74]. In a study of 68 LVHT patients mutations in the LMNA gene were found in 5% of the cases but of the 68 patients only 2 patients had an NMD [76].

AMPD1

AMPD1 encodes for the myo-adenylate deaminase, an enzyme involved in deamination of AMP molecules. *AMPD1* has a widespread expression, particularly in type-I muscle fibers, smooth muscle fibers, and in neurons. Mutations in AMPD1 may be asymptomatic, may cause myalgias, rhabdomyolysis, or metabolic myopathy, manifesting with fatigue, cramps, muscle pain, or recurrent myoglobinurea. *AMPD1* variants have been associated with coronary heart disease or heart failure. Only in a single patient with AMPD1 associated myopathy has LVHT been reported [20]. The patient was a 53 years old male presenting with easy fatigability, myalgias since boyhood, and recurrently elevated creatine-kinase [20]. Holter-ECG showed nocturnal sinus-bradycardia and echocardiography showed myocardial thickening in addition to LVHT [20]. LVHT was confirmed by cardiac MRI.

MYH7

MYH7 encodes for the beta-myosin heavy chain, a sarcomeric protein predominantly expressed in the skeletal muscle and the myocardium. It mainly occurs in slow-twitch fibers (type-I-fibers). Mutations in *MYH7* were identified in patients with HCM, DCM, Laing distal myopathy, myosin storage myopathy, and axial myopathy (dropped head, camptocormia) [77]. Only in single patients have *MYH7* mutations been reported in patients with myopathy and LVHT simultaneously [23, 24, 77]. Myopathy together with LVHT was first described by Ruggiero et al. in 2013 [24]. In this study, three members of an Italian family presented with Laing-like distal myopathy and LVHT. Muscle biopsy showed fiber-type disproportion. Mild distal myopathy was also reported in a female with LVHT carrying a *MYH7* mutation [23]. Other members of the index patient's family presented with myopathy plus anginal chest pain, impaired relaxation, or DCM [23]. In a cohort of 21 Italian patients with MYH7 myopathy, 5 had LVHT [77]. It has not been reported if the 3 previously reported Italian patients [24] were included in this cohort or not.

More frequently than mutation carriers with LVHT plus NMD, patients with LVHT and a *MYH7* mutation but without neurological investigation have been reported. In a study of 190 patients with LVHT from the USA, 8 were found to carry a *MYH7* variant. Though cardiologists did not report muscle symptoms, it remains unknown if any of the included patients manifested also in the skeletal muscle [39]. This uncertainty remains since the patients were not systematically referred to the neurologist and since these patients obviously had not exhibited muscular manifestations [39]. In a study of 102 patients with LVHT, *MYH7* mutations were detected in 19 of them [58]. Unfortunately, these patients were not systematically referred for neuromuscular evaluation. In a study of 57 Chinese patients with LVHT, 6 carried a mutation in the *MYH7* gene [78].

CNBP/ZNF9

CNBP/ZNF9 encodes for a protein of which the function is unknown but which is mainly expressed in the heart and muscle. Intron-1 of the gene contains the complex repeat motif $(TG)_n(TSGT)_n(CCTG)_n$. Expansion of this motif between >75 and up to 11,000 repeats causes myotonic dystrophy type-2 (MD2). MD2 is a multisystem disorder manifesting mainly in the muscle, eyes, and endocrine organs. Most patients present with myotonia, cataract, diabetes, and elevated, follicle stimulating hormone. Cardiac involvement may occur and includes ventricular arrhythmias and DCM [79]. Only in a single patient with MD2 has LVHT been reported so far [26]. This was a 61 years male with DCM and apical hypertrabeculation [26]. Additionally, the patient presented with hand myotonia and progressive limb muscle weakness evolving for >20 years. He also had diabetes mellitus and an isolated elevation of gamma-glutamyl transpeptidase [26].

GLA

GLA encodes for alpha-galactosidase, an enzyme which cleaves the terminal galactose from ceramide trihexoside. Mutations in the gene result in accumulation of ceramide trihexoside in neurons, ganglia, myocardiocytes, kidney, and the smooth muscle cells. The phenotype of alpha-galactosidase deficiency is known as Fabry's disease, of which the severity correlates with the residual enzyme activity, being 1–17%. Cardiac involvement in Fabry's disease includes HCM, conduction defects, ectasia of arteries, and myocardial infarction. LVHT has been reported in Fabry's disease only once so far. A 32 years old female was found to carry a *GLA* mutation upon a family screening. She did not manifest clinically with the disease but echocardiography revealed typical hypertrabeculation of the mid-ventricular and the apical segments of the left ventricular myocardium [29].

RYR1

RYR1 encodes for the ryanodine receptor-1, also known as skeletal muscle calcium release channel or skeletal muscle-type ryanodine receptor. The gene is mainly expressed in the skeletal muscle. Mutations in RYR1 manifest phenotypically heterogeneously as multiminicore myopathy, atypical periodic paralysis, distal myopathy, centronuclear myopathy, central core disease, arthrogryposis multiplex congenital, or as malignant hyperthermia susceptibility. Cardiac disease in carriers of RYR1 mutations is rare despite expression of *RYR1* also in cardiomyocytes [80]. SCD has been reported in patients with malignant hyperthermia susceptibility due to *RYR1* mutations. Only a single patient with multiminicore myopathy due to a *RYR1* mutation has been reported in whom also LVHT was detected [36]. The patient was a 16 years old Turkish male with myopathic face, weakness and hypotonia of the limb muscles with proximal predominance, and hyperlordosis [36]. Electromyography was myopathic and muscle biopsy showed multiminicore myopathy [36]. Echocardiography showed slightly enlarged cardiac cavities, mildly reduced ejection fraction, and typical LVHT of the apex [36].

MYH7B

The *MYH7B* gene belongs to the *MYH* gene family, which, in humans, also includes the *MYH6* and *MYH7* genes, both clustered on chromosome 14 [35]. The *MYH7B* gene encodes for the myosin heavy chain 7B, which is particularly expressed in the skeletal and the cardiac muscle [35]. Very low expression was observed in the brain, testes, ovary, liver, and blood [35]. Mutations in the *MYH7B* gene have been only rarely reported. In a single Italian family, a *MYH7B* mutation manifested in the skeletal muscle as congenital fiber type disproportion [35]. In four of the family members screening for cardiac involvement revealed LVHT. The 10 year old index patient presented with myopathy manifesting with proximal muscle weakness, scoliosis, and amyotrophy. She had a history of hypotonia, poor sucking, and persistent crying since birth. Persistent arterial duct and patent foramen ovale resolved spontaneously [35]. In addition to LVHT, the index case presented with long-QT, myocardial thickening, repolarisation abnormalities, and reduced systolic function [35]. Interestingly, the index patient additionally carried a mutation in the *ITGA7* gene [35], which, however, was not made responsible for the phenotype. Other patients with myopathy and LVHT due to a mutation in the *MYH7B* gene have not been reported.

LAMP2

LAMP2 encodes for the lysosome-associated membrane glycoprotein-2. LAMP2 provides selectins with carbohydrate ligands and plays a role in the protection, maintenance, and adhesion of the lysosome and possibly also in tumour cell metastasis. Mutations in the *LAMP2* gene cause Danon disease, also known as glycogen storage disease IIb, an X-linked lysosomal glycogen storage disorder, which is clinically characterised by HCM, myopathy, and intellectual decline. LVHT in Danon disease has been reported only in a single patient so far. The patient was a 19 years old mildly mentally retarded male in whom LVHT was detected after a syncope during a basketball game at age 14 years [36]. At age of 16 year, he developed heart failure. Despite immediate treatment, heart failure became intractable and the patient underwent heart transplantation. For immunosuppression he received tacrolimus, daclicumab, prednisone, and mycophenolate mofetil. After transfer to the ward, the patient developed muscle weakness why he underwent muscle biopsy. Upon muscle biopsy, Danon disease was suspected and sequencing of the *LAMP2* gene revealed a causative mutation [36].

TTN

The *TTN* gene is the largest of the human genes so far detected. It encodes for titin, a giant protein, which is mainly expressed in the striated muscles and cardiac muscle [40]. Mutations in the *TTN* gene manifest with marked phenotypic heterogeneity. Heterozygous *TTN* truncating mutations have been reported as a major cause of dominant DCM, HCM, cardiac septal defects, isolated LVHT, Emery-Dreifuss muscular dystrophy, distal myopathy, or arthrogryposis [40]. However, relatively few *TTN* mutations and phenotypes are known, and the pathophysiological role of titin in cardiac and skeletal muscle conditions is incompletely understood. Myopathy plus LVHT has been reported in a single family carrying a *TTN* mutation so far [40]. In a study of 190 patients with LVHT, a *TTN* mutation was detected in 14 of them [39]. In a three-generation family with autosomal dominant CMP due to a *TTN* mutation, LVHT was detected in 7 family members [41]. In a single child with bradycardia and LVHT, mutations in the *RYR2, CASQ2,* and *TTN* gene respectively were discovered, [42]. In the latter three studies it is unclear if these LVHT patients had been investigated for NMD.

PLEC1

PLEC1 encodes for plectin, a linker protein involved in cytoskeletal organisation, which is particularly expressed in epithelia, skeletal muscle, and myocardium [47]. *PLEC1* mutations manifest phenotypically with broad heterogeneity, including epidermiolysis bullosa simplex (EBS), EBS plus muscular dystrophy, and pyloric atresia. EBS plus muscular dystrophy is characterised by skin fragility and late-onset muscular dystrophy, but significant phenotypic heterogeneity can occur [47]. Even the dermatological manifestations vary regarding severity and include neonatal skin fragility and mucosal vulnerability resulting in tracheal and urethral tract complications [47]. Muscular dystrophy is similarly variable in onset and severity, characterised by diffuse limb muscle weakness with onset between infancy and 4th decade of life. LVHT has been reported only in a single carrier of a *PLEC1* mutation [47]. This was an 18 years old Afro-American male with blistering at the elbows at birth, being subsequently diagnosed as EBS. Developmental delay and first muscular manifestations were observed at age of 2 years [47]. By age of 4 years, the patient had lost the ability to rise from the floor and to walk stairs independently [47]. Since age of 10 years, he was wheel-chair bound. Work-up for cardiac involvement an age17 years by cMRI revealed LVHT.

POMPT2

POMPT2, together with POMPT1, encodes for the protein-O-manosyl-transferase, which is involved in the glycosylation of alpha-dystroglycan [49]. Hypoglycosilation of alpha-dystroglycan results in dystroglycanopathies of which Walker-Warburg syndrome (WWS) is the most severe. WWS is a rare autosomal recessive congenital muscular dystrophy (CMD) clinically characterised by eye and brain abnormalities. WWS is genetically heterogeneous and may not only be caused by POMPT2 mutations but also by mutations in the FKTN, FKRP, POMGnT1, POMGnT2, ISPD, B3GNT1, or LARGE1 genes respectively [49]. Cardiac involvement is infrequent in WWS [81]. Only 1 WWS patient with coarctation of the aorta has been reported. The only patient in whom LVHT has been reported so far was a neonate with facial dysmorphism (hypertelorism, low set ears, frontal bossing, micro-retrognathia), laterally displaced nipples, hypospadias, and muscle hypotonia [49]. ECG in this patient showed incomplete left bundle branch block, left ventricular hypertrophy, and T-wave inversion. Echocardiography revealed an atrial septal defect, shunting left-to-right, a muscular ventricular septal defect, and LVHT [49]. At an age of 4 months the patient experienced a cardiogenic shock due to congestive heart failure and recurrent episodes of cardiac arrest, the last one being unresponsive to resuscitation. Heart failure and conduction defects were attributed to LVHT [49].

Diagnostic Work-Up of NCCM

For a comprehensive diagnostic work-up, we refer to Chap. 2 of this title.

LVHT or NCCM is usually diagnosed accidentally on echocardiography [82]. In the young age group, patients are usually referred for syncopes or palpitations whereas in the older age groups patients are usually referred for heart failure [82]. However, there are groups of patients at risk having LVHT in a higher frequency than the general population. These risk groups include patients with chromosomal defects, NMD, black Africans, pregnant females, and athletes. This is why patients of these at-risk groups need to be systematically investigated for LVHT and, vice versa, patients with LVHT require work up for chromosomal defects and NMDs. A shortcoming in the work-up of patients with LVHT, however, is that often they are not investigated for associated non-cardiac disease or the genetic background. Since NMDs are frequently only mildly manifesting or even subclinical, neurologists specialised in NMDs need to be involved. For cardiologists who diagnose LVHT, neuromuscular features are frequently not evident why the NMD often goes undetected. For this reason, all patients with LVHT should be seen by a neurologist. Vice versa, all patients with an NMD should be referred to the cardiologist as soon as the diagnosis is established or even when it is suspected, to assess if cardiac involvement is present and if the patient requires cardiac therapy. Diagnosing the NMD in a LVHT patient may be challenging since the NMD may be absent, subclinical, or only mildly manifesting. In these cases, the NMD may be easily overlooked, particularly if the patient was not thoroughly investigated. Why mutations in certain genes manifest with or without NMD is poorly understood. An example for the variable expression is the *LMNA* gene. LVHT has been repeatedly reported in patients carrying *LMNA* mutations [18, 19, 75], but only in a few patients LGMD has been reported.

Treatment of NCCM

For a comprehensive overview, we refer to Chaps. 5, 6 and 9 of this title.

Treatment of LVHT in patients with an NMD is not at variance compared to patients with LVHT but without an NMD. LVHT is asymptomatic in the majority of the cases but may be complicated by intertrabecular thrombus formation leading to cardiac thombo-embolism, heart failure, or ventricular arrhythmias, potentially leading to SCD. Primary prevention of cardio-embolism by oral anticoagulation is not indicated in patients with asymptomatic LVHT plus an NMD. However, if LVHT is associated with severe heart failure, or atrial fibrillation, oral anticoagulation is indicated. Oral anticoagulation should be also applied for secondary prevention of cardiac thrombo-embolism if a LVHT patient has a previous history of stroke/embolism. Heart failure in LVHT with NMD requires the same established therapy as heart failure in other patients (i.e. ACE-inhibitors, beta-blockers, diuretics). In case malignant ventricular arrhythmias are detected, implantation of an implantable cardioverter defibrillator (ICD) should be considered. To detect ventricular arrhythmias in LVHT patients with an NMD, either repeated 24-h or longer Holter recordings are necessary. In case of unclear clinical presentation, implantation of a reveal-recorder should be considered. If implantation of an ICD is indicated but not immediately feasible, application of a wearable cardioverter defibrillator should be recommended. Primary and secondary prevention of malignant ventricular arrhythmias is achieved by implantation of an ICD.

Outcome

There are only few studies available investigating the outcome of NMD patients with LVHT. In a study of 220 LVHT patients of whom 134 had a NMD, predictors of mortality on multivariate analysis were increased age, heart failure, atrial fibrillation, bradycardia, and presence of a NMD [72]. Thus, presence of an NMD in LVHT patients seems to have a strong impact on the outcome of these patients.

Conclusions

NCCM or LVHT is a morphological cardiac abnormality associated with an increased risk of intraventricular thrombus formation, heart failure, and ventricular arrhythmias with SCD. LVHT has a low prevalence in the general population but an increased prevalence among patients with a NMD and chromosomal defects.

Among these groups, LVHT is most prevalent in NMDs. LVHT may occur in some patients with a certain NMD type but not in the majority of the patients. Also, in LVHT patients with a certain mutated gene only some will manifest also with a NMD. Though LVHT has been reported in association with a number of mutated genes, which manifest as pure NMD or NMD with multiorgan disease, a causal relation has not been established yet since these mutations have been also described in association with an NMD but without LVHT. These genes include *DMD, TAZ, DTNA, mtDNA genes (ND1, tRNA(Leu), COX3, ND4), LDB3, DMPK, LMNA, AMPD1, PMP22, MYH7, CNBP, GLA, RYR1, DNAJC19, MYH7B, LAMP2, TTN, GARS, SDHD, HADHB, PLEC1, MIPEP*, and *POMPT2*. A causal relation between mutations in these genes and the occurrence is rather unlikely since only a limited number of patients carrying these mutations present with LVHT, since mutations in many different genes cause the same morphological abnormality, and since a causal relation between any of these mutations and LVHT has not been proven yet. Since LVHT is associated with complications, it is essential to detect the abnormality, to monitor it adequately, and to initiate adequate measures when indicated. Thus, all patients with an NMD need to be prospectively investigated for LVHT, and all patients with LVHT need to be prospectively investigated for NMD. Concerning the primary prevention of complications from LVHT, no consensus has been reached so far. Detection of an associated genetic defect in a patient with LVHT does not alter cardiac therapy but may influence the symptomatic treatment of the neuromuscular manifestations. Thus, it is nonetheless useful to test LVHT patients for concomitant genetic defects, despite absence of a causal relation between LVHT and any of the so far detected genetic defects associated with LVHT. There is a general need to encourage and conduct studies about the prevalence of LVHT in different NMDs worldwide and about the pathogenetic relation between NMDs and LVHT.

Acknowledgements None

Conflicts of Interest There are no conflicts of interest.

No funding was received.

References

1. Finsterer J. Cardio genetics, neurogenetics, and pathogenetics of left ventricular hypertrabeculation/noncompaction. Pediatr Cardiol. 2009;30:659–81.
2. Stöllberger C, Finsterer J, Blazek G, Bittner RE. Left ventricular non-compaction in a patient with Becker's muscular dystrophy. Heart. 1996;76:380.
3. Kimura K, Takenaka K, Ebihara A, Uno K, Morita H, Nakajima T, Ozawa T, Aida I, Yonemochi Y, Higuchi S, Motoyoshi Y, Mikata T, Uchida I, Ishihara T, Komori T, Kitao R, Nagata T, Takeda S, Yatomi Y, Nagai R, Komuro I. Prognostic impact of left ventricular noncompaction in patients with Duchenne/Becker muscular dystrophy–prospective multicenter cohort study. Int J Cardiol. 2013;168:1900–4.
4. Bleyl SB, Mumford BR, Thompson V, Carey JC, Pysher TJ, Chin TK, Ward K. Neonatal, lethal noncompaction of the left ventricular myocardium is allelic with Barth syndrome. Am J Hum Genet. 1997;61:868–72.

5. Finsterer J, Stöllberger C. Hypertrabeculated left ventricle in mitochondriopathy. Heart. 1998;80:632.
6. Ichida F, Tsubata S, Bowles KR, Haneda N, Uese K, Miyawaki T, Dreyer WJ, Messina J, Li H, Bowles NE, Towbin JA. Novel gene mutations in patients with left ventricular noncompaction or Barth syndrome. Circulation. 2001;103:1256–63.
7. Xing Y, Ichida F, Matsuoka T, Isobe T, Ikemoto Y, Higaki T, Tsuji T, Haneda N, Kuwabara A, Chen R, Futatani T, Tsubata S, Watanabe S, Watanabe K, Hirono K, Uese K, Miyawaki T, Bowles KR, Bowles NE, Towbin JA. Genetic analysis in patients with left ventricular noncompaction and evidence for genetic heterogeneity. Mol Genet Metab. 2006;88:71–7.
8. Finsterer J, Stöllberger C, Kopsa W. Noncompaction on cardiac MRI in a patient with nail-patella syndrome and mitochondriopathy. Cardiology. 2003;100:48–9.
9. Vatta M, Mohapatra B, Jimenez S, Sanchez X, Faulkner G, Perles Z, Sinagra G, Lin JH, Vu TM, Zhou Q, Bowles KR, Di Lenarda A, Schimmenti L, Fox M, Chrisco MA, Murphy RT, McKenna W, Elliott P, Bowles NE, Chen J, Valle G, Towbin JA. Mutations in Cypher/ZASP in patients with dilated cardiomyopathy and left ventricular non-compaction. J Am Coll Cardiol. 2003;42:2014–27.
10. Xi Y, Ai T, De Lange E, Li Z, Wu G, Brunelli L, Kyle WB, Turker I, Cheng J, Ackerman MJ, Kimura A, Weiss JN, Qu Z, Kim JJ, Faulkner G, Vatta M. Loss of function of hNav1.5 by a ZASP1 mutation associated with intraventricular conduction disturbances in left ventricular noncompaction. Circ Arrhythm Electrophysiol. 2012;5:1017–26.
11. Hachiya A, Motoki N, Akazawa Y, Matsuzaki S, Hirono K, Hata Y, Nishida N, Ichida F, Koike K. Left ventricular non-compaction revealed by aortic regurgitation due to Kawasaki disease in a boy with LDB3 mutation. Pediatr Int. 2016;58:797–800.
12. Stöllberger C, Winkler-Dworak M, Blazek G, Finsterer J. Left ventricular hypertrabeculation/noncompaction with and without neuromuscular disorders. Int J Cardiol. 2004;97:89–92.
13. Choudhary P, Nandakumar R, Greig H, Broadhurst P, Dean J, Puranik R, Celermajer DS, Hillis GS. Structural and electrical cardiac abnormalities are prevalent in asymptomatic adults with myotonic dystrophy. Heart. 2016;102:1472–8.
14. Finsterer J, Stöllberger C, Wegmann R, Janssen LA. Acquired left ventricular hypertrabeculation/noncompaction in myotonic dystrophy type 1. Int J Cardiol. 2009;137:310–3.
15. Sá MI, Cabral S, Costa PD, Coelho T, Freitas M, Torres S, Gomes JL. Cardiac involveent in type 1 myotonic dystrophy. Rev Port Cardiol. 2007;26:829–40.
16. Finsterer J, Stöllberger C, Kopsa W, Jaksch M. Wolff-Parkinson-White syndrome and isolated left ventricular abnormal trabeculation as a manifestation of Leber's hereditary optic neuropathy. Can J Cardiol. 2001;17:464–6.
17. Finsterer J, Stöllberger C, Michaela J. Familial left ventricular hypertrabeculation in two blind brothers. Cardiovasc Pathol. 2002;11:146–8.
18. Hermida-Prieto M, Monserrat L, Castro-Beiras A, Laredo R, Soler R, Peteiro J, Rodríguez E, Bouzas B, Alvarez N, Muñiz J, Crespo-Leiro M. Familial dilated cardiomyopathy and isolated left ventricular noncompaction associated with lamin A/C gene mutations. Am J Cardiol. 2004;94:50–4.
19. Liu Z, Shan H, Huang J, Li N, Hou C, Pu J. A novel lamin A/C gene missense mutation (445 V > E) in immunoglobulin-like fold associated with left ventricular non-compaction. Europace. 2016;18:617–22.
20. Finsterer J, Schoser B, Stöllberger C. Myoadenylate-deaminase gene mutation associated with left ventricular hypertrabeculation/non-compaction. Acta Cardiol. 2004;59:453–6.
21. Finsterer J, Gelpi E, Stöllberger C. Left ventricular hypertrabeculation/noncompaction as a cardiac manifestation of Duchenne muscular dystrophy under non-invasive positive-pressure ventilation. Acta Cardiol. 2005;60:445–8.
22. Corrado G, Checcarelli N, Santarone M, Stollberger C, Finsterer J. Left ventricular hypertrabeculation/noncompaction with PMP22 duplication-based Charcot-Marie-Tooth disease type 1A. Cardiology. 2006;105:142–5.
23. Finsterer J, Brandau O, Stöllberger C, Wallefeld W, Laing NG, Laccone F. Distal myosin heavy chain-7 myopathy due to the novel transition c.5566G>A (p.E1856K) with high interfamilial cardiac variability and putative anticipation. Neuromuscul Disord. 2014;24:721–5.

24. Ruggiero L, Fiorillo C, Gibertini S, De Stefano F, Manganelli F, Iodice R, Vitale F, Zanotti S, Galderisi M, Mora M, Santoro L. A rare mutation in MYH7 gene occurs with overlapping phenotype. Biochem Biophys Res Commun. 2015;457:262–6.
25. Alter P, Maisch B. Non-compaction cardiomyopathy in an adult with hereditary spherocytosis. Eur J Heart Fail. 2007;9:98–9.
26. Wahbi K, Meune C, Bassez G, Laforêt P, Vignaux O, Marmursztejn J, Bécane HM, Eymard B, Duboc D. Left ventricular non-compaction in a patient with myotonic dystrophy type 2. Neuromuscul Disord. 2008;18:331–3.
27. Thevathasan W, Squier W, MacIver DH, Hilton DA, Fathers E, Hilton-Jones D. Oculopharyngodistal myopathy–a possible association with cardiomyopathy. Neuromuscul Disord. 2011;21:121–5.
28. Lee YC, Chang CJ, Bali D, Chen YT, Yan YT. Glycogen-branching enzyme deficiency leads to abnormal cardiac development: novel insights into glycogen storage disease IV. Hum Mol Genet. 2011;20:455–65.
29. Azevedo O, Gaspar P, Sá Miranda C, Cunha D, Medeiros R, Lourenço A. Left ventricular noncompaction in a patient with fabry disease: overdiagnosis, morphological manifestation of fabry disease or two unrelated rare conditions in the same patient. Cardiology. 2011;119:155–9.
30. Martins E, Pinho T, Carpenter S, Leite S, Garcia R, Madureira A, Oliveira JP. Histopathological evidence of Fabry disease in a female patient with left ventricular noncompaction. Rev Port Cardiol. 2014;33:565.e1–6.
31. Finsterer J, Stöllberger C, Vlckova Z, Gencik M. On the edge of noncompaction: minimally manifesting Duchenne carrier due to the dystrophin mutation n.2867A>C. Int J Cardiol. 2013;165:e18–20.
32. Şimşek Z, Açar G, Akçakoyun M, Esen Ö, Emiroğlu Y, Esen AM. Left ventricular noncompaction in a patient with multiminicore disease. J Cardiovasc Med. 2012;13:660–2.
33. Cosson L, Toutain A, Simard G, Kulik W, Matyas G, Guichet A, Blasco H, Maakaroun-Vermesse Z, Vaillant MC, Le Caignec C, Chantepie A, Labarthe F. Barth syndrome in a female patient. Mol Genet Metab. 2012;106:115–20.
34. Ojala T, Polinati P, Manninen T, Hiippala A, Rajantie J, Karikoski R, Suomalainen A, Tyni T. New mutation of mitochondrial DNAJC19 causing dilated and noncompaction cardiomyopathy, anemia, ataxia, and male genital anomalies. Pediatr Res. 2012;72:432–7.
35. Esposito T, Sampaolo S, Limongelli G, Varone A, Formicola D, Diodato D, Farina O, Napolitano F, Pacileo G, Gianfrancesco F, Di Iorio G. Digenic mutational inheritance of the integrin alpha 7 and the myosin heavy chain 7B genes causes congenital myopathy with left ventricular non-compact cardiomyopathy. Orphanet J Rare Dis. 2013;8:91. https://doi.org/10.1186/1750-1172-8-91.
36. Van Der Starre P, Deuse T, Pritts C, Brun C, Vogel H, Oyer P. Late profound muscle weakness following heart transplantation due to Danon disease. Muscle Nerve. 2013;47:135–7.
37. Liu S, Bai Y, Huang J, Zhao H, Zhang X, Hu S, Wei Y. Do mitochondria contribute to left ventricular non-compaction cardiomyopathy? New findings from myocardium of patients with left ventricular non-compaction cardiomyopathy. Mol Genet Metab. 2013;109:100–6.
38. Wang J, Zhu Q, Kong X, Hu B, Shi H, Liang B, Zhou M, Cao F. A combination of left ventricular hypertrabeculation/noncompaction and muscular dystrophy in a stroke patient. Int J Cardiol. 2014;174:e68–71.
39. Miszalski-Jamka K, Jefferies JL, Mazur W, Głowacki J, Hu J, Lazar M, Gibbs RA, Liczko J, Kłyś J, Venner E, Muzny DM, Rycaj J, Białkowski J, Kluczewska E, Kalarus Z, Jhangiani S, Al-Khalidi H, Kukulski T, Lupski JR, Craigen WJ, Bainbridge MN. Novel genetic triggers and genotype-phenotype correlations in patients with left ventricular noncompaction. Circ Cardiovasc Genet. 2017;10:e001763. https://doi.org/10.1161/CIRCGENETICS.117.001763.
40. Chauveau C, Bonnemann CG, Julien C, Kho AL, Marks H, Talim B, Maury P, Arne-Bes MC, Uro-Coste E, Alexandrovich A, Vihola A, Schafer S, Kaufmann B, Medne L, Hübner N, Foley AR, Santi M, Udd B, Topaloglu H, Moore SA, Gotthardt M, Samuels ME, Gautel M, Ferreiro A. Recessive TTN truncating mutations define novel forms of core myopathy with heart disease. Hum Mol Genet. 2014;23:980–91.

41. Hastings R, de Villiers CP, Hooper C, Ormondroyd L, Pagnamenta A, Lise S, Salatino S, Knight SJ, Taylor JC, Thomson KL, Arnold L, Chatziefthimiou SD, Konarev PV, Wilmanns M, Ehler E, Ghisleni A, Gautel M, Blair E, Watkins H, Gehmlich K. Combination of whole genome sequencing, linkage, and functional studies implicates a missense mutation in titin as a cause of autosomal dominant cardiomyopathy with features of left ventricular noncompaction. Circ Cardiovasc Genet. 2016;9:426–35.
42. Egan KR, Ralphe JC, Weinhaus L, Maginot KR. Just sinus bradycardia or something more serious? Case Rep Pediatr. 2013;2013:736164. https://doi.org/10.1155/2013/736164.
43. McMillan HJ, Schwartzentruber J, Smith A, Lee S, Chakraborty P, Bulman DE, Beaulieu CL, Majewski J, Boycott KM, Geraghty MT. Compound heterozygous mutations in glycyl-tRNA synthetase are a proposed cause of systemic mitochondrial disease. BMC Med Genet. 2014;15:36.
44. Alston CL, Ceccatelli Berti C, Blakely EL, Oláhová M, He L, McMahon CJ, Olpin SE, Hargreaves IP, Nolli C, McFarland R, Goffrini P, O'Sullivan MJ, Taylor RW. A recessive homozygous p.Asp92Gly SDHD mutation causes prenatal cardiomyopathy and a severe mitochondrial complex II deficiency. Hum Genet. 2015;134:869–79.
45. Jain-Ghai S, Cameron JM, Al Maawali A, Blaser S, MacKay N, Robinson B, Raiman J. Complex II deficiency–a case report and review of the literature. Am J Med Genet A. 2013;161A:285–94.
46. Ojala T, Nupponen I, Saloranta C, Sarkola T, Sekar P, Breilin A, Tyni T. Fetal left ventricular noncompaction cardiomyopathy and fatal outcome due to complete deficiency of mitochondrial trifunctional protein. Eur J Pediatr. 2015;174:1689–92.
47. Villa CR, Ryan TD, Collins JJ, Taylor MD, Lucky AW, Jefferies JL. Left ventricular non-compaction cardiomyopathy associated with epidermolysis bullosa simplex with muscular dystrophy and PLEC1 mutation. Neuromuscul Disord. 2015;25:165–8.
48. Eldomery MK, Akdemir ZC, Vögtle FN, Charng WL, Mulica P, Rosenfeld JA, Gambin T, Gu S, Burrage LC, Al Shamsi A, Penney S, Jhangiani SN, Zimmerman HH, Muzny DM, Wang X, Tang J, Medikonda R, Ramachandran PV, Wong LJ, Boerwinkle E, Gibbs RA, Eng CM, Lalani SR, Hertecant J, Rodenburg RJ, Abdul-Rahman OA, Yang Y, Xia F, Wang MC, Lupski JR, Meisinger C, Sutton VR. MIPEP recessive variants cause a syndrome of left ventricular non-compaction, hypotonia, and infantile death. Genome Med. 2016;8:106.
49. Abdullah S, Hawkins C, Wilson G, Yoon G, Mertens L, Carter MT, Guerin A. Noncompaction cardiomyopathy in an infant with Walker-Warburg syndrome. Am J Med Genet A. 2017;173:3082–6.
50. Budde BS, Binner P, Waldmüller S, Höhne W, Blankenfeldt W, Hassfeld S, Brömsen J, Dermintzoglou A, Wieczorek M, May E, Kirst E, Selignow C, Rackebrandt K, Müller M, Goody RS, Vosberg HP, Nürnberg P, Scheffold T. Noncompaction of the ventricular myocardium is associated with a de novo mutation in the beta-myosin heavy chain gene. PLoS One. 2007;2:e1362.
51. Mavrogeni SI, Markousis-Mavrogenis G, Papavasiliou A, Papadopoulos G, Kolovou G. Cardiac involvement in Duchenne muscular dystrophy and related dystrophinopathies. Methods Mol Biol. 2018;1687:31–42.
52. Finsterer J, Stöllberger C, Wexberg P, Schukro C. Left ventricular hypertrabeculation/noncompaction in a Duchenne/Becker muscular dystrophy carrier with epilepsy. Int J Cardiol. 2012;162:e3–5.
53. Statile CJ, Taylor MD, Mazur W, Cripe LH, King E, Pratt J, Benson DW, Hor KN. Left ventricular noncompaction in Duchenne muscular dystrophy. J Cardiovasc Magn Reson. 2013;15:67. https://doi.org/10.1186/1532-429X-15-67.
54. Schelhorn J, Schoenecker A, Neudorf U, Schemuth H, Nensa F, Nassenstein K, Forsting M, Schara U, Schlosser T. Cardiac pathologies in female carriers of Duchenne muscular dystrophy assessed by cardiovascular magnetic resonance imaging. Eur Radiol. 2015;25:3066–72.
55. Ferreira C, Thompson R, Vernon H. Barth syndrome. In: Adam MP, Ardinger HH, Pagon RA, Wallace SE, LJH B, Stephens K, Amemiya A, editors. GeneReviews®. Seattle: University of Washington; 2014.

56. Ronvelia D, Greenwood J, Platt J, Hakim S, Zaragoza MV. Intrafamilial variability for novel TAZ gene mutation: Barth syndrome with dilated cardiomyopathy and heart failure in an infant and left ventricular noncompaction in his great-uncle. Mol Genet Metab. 2012;107:428–32.
57. Thiels C, Fleger M, Huemer M, Rodenburg RJ, Vaz FM, Houtkooper RH, Haack TB, Prokisch H, Feichtinger RG, Lücke T, Mayr JA, Wortmann SB. Atypical clinical presentations of TAZ mutations: an underdiagnosed cause of growth retardation? JIMD Rep. 2016;29:89–93.
58. Wang C, Hata Y, Hirono K, Takasaki A, Ozawa SW, Nakaoka H, Saito K, Miyao N, Okabe M, Ibuki K, Nishida N, Origasa H, Yu X, Bowles NE, Ichida F, LVNC Study Collaborators. A Wide and specific spectrum of genetic variants and genotype-phenotype correlations revealed by next-generation sequencing in patients with left ventricular noncompaction. J Am Heart Assoc. 2017;6(9):e006210. https://doi.org/10.1161/JAHA.117.006210.
59. Pignatelli RH, McMahon CJ, Dreyer WJ, Denfield SW, Price J, Belmont JW, Craigen WJ, Wu J, El Said H, Bezold LI, Clunie S, Fernbach S, Bowles NE, Towbin JA. Clinical characterization of left ventricular noncompaction in children: a relatively common form of cardiomyopathy. Circulation. 2003;108:2672–8.
60. Spencer CT, Bryant RM, Day J, Gonzalez IL, Colan SD, Thompson WR, Berthy J, Redfearn SP, Byrne BJ. Cardiac and clinical phenotype in Barth syndrome. Pediatrics. 2006;118:e337–46.
61. Cao Q, Shen Y, Liu X, Yu X, Yuan P, Wan R, Liu X, Peng X, He W, Pu J, Hong K. Phenotype and functional analyses in a transgenic mouse model of left ventricular noncompaction caused by a DTNA mutation. Int Heart J. 2017;58:939–47.
62. Tang S, Batra A, Zhang Y, Ebenroth ES, Huang T. Left ventricular noncompaction is associated with mutations in the mitochondrial genome. Mitochondrion. 2010;10:350–7.
63. Zarrouk Mahjoub S, Mehri S, Ourda F, Boussaada R, Mechmeche R, Arab SB, Finsterer J. Transition m.3308T>C in the ND1 gene is associated with left ventricular hypertrabeculation/noncompaction. Cardiology. 2011;118:153–8.
64. Limongelli G, Tome-Esteban M, Dejthevaporn C, Rahman S, Hanna MG, Elliott PM. Prevalence and natural history of heart disease in adults with primary mitochondrial respiratory chain disease. Eur J Heart Fail. 2010;12:114–21.
65. Finsterer J, Stöllberger C, Steger C, Cozzarini W. Complete heart block associated with noncompaction, nail-patella syndrome, and mitochondrial myopathy. J Electrocardiol. 2007;40:352–4.
66. MIPEP. Wikipedia. https://en.wikipedia.org/wiki/MIPEP. Accessed Jan 2018.
67. Davili Z, Johar S, Hughes C, Kveselis D, Hoo J. Succinate dehydrogenase deficiency associated with dilated cardiomyopathy and ventricular noncompaction. Eur J Pediatr. 2007;166:867–70.
68. Wang J, Kong X, Han P, Hu B, Cao F, Liu Y, Zhu Q. Combination of mitochondrial myopathy and biventricular hypertrabeculation/noncompaction. Neuromuscul Disord. 2016;26:165–9.
69. Scaglia F, Towbin JA, Craigen WJ, Belmont JW, Smith EO, Neish SR, Ware SM, Hunter JV, Fernbach SD, Vladutiu GD, Wong LJ, Vogel H. Clinical spectrum, morbidity, and mortality in 113 pediatric patients with mitochondrial disease. Pediatrics. 2004;114:925–31.
70. Yaplito-Lee J, Weintraub R, Jamsen K, Chow CW, Thorburn DR, Boneh A. Cardiac manifestations in oxidative phosphorylation disorders of childhood. J Pediatr. 2007;150:407–11.
71. Dhar R, Reardon W, McMahon CJ. Biventricular non-compaction hypertrophic cardiomyopathy in association with congenital complete heart block and type I mitochondrial complex deficiency. Cardiol Young. 2015;25:1019–21.
72. Stöllberger C, Blazek G, Gessner M, Bichler K, Wegner C, Finsterer J. Neuromuscular comorbidity, heart failure, and atrial fibrillation as prognostic factors in left ventricular hypertrabeculation/noncompaction. Herz. 2015;40:906–11.
73. Worman HJ. Cell signaling abnormalities in cardiomyopathy caused by lamin A/C gene mutations. Biochem Soc Trans. 2017;46(1):37–42. https://doi.org/10.1042/BST20170236.
74. Rankin J, Auer-Grumbach M, Bagg W, Colclough K, Nguyen TD, Fenton-May J, Hattersley A, Hudson J, Jardine P, Josifova D, Longman C, McWilliam R, Owen K, Walker M, Wehnert M, Ellard S. Extreme phenotypic diversity and nonpenetrance in families with the LMNA gene mutation R644C. Am J Med Genet A. 2008;146A:1530–42.

75. Parent JJ, Towbin JA, Jefferies JL. Left ventricular noncompaction in a family with lamin A/C gene mutation. Tex Heart Inst J. 2015;42:73–6.
76. Sedaghat-Hamedani F, Haas J, Zhu F, Geier C, Kayvanpour E, Liss M, Lai A, Frese K, Pribe-Wolferts R, Amr A, Li DT, Samani OS, Carstensen A, Bordalo DM, Müller M, Fischer C, Shao J, Wang J, Nie M, Yuan L, Haßfeld S, Schwartz C, Zhou M, Zhou Z, Shu Y, Wang M, Huang K, Zeng Q, Cheng L, Fehlmann T, Ehlermann P, Keller A, Dieterich C, Streckfuß-Bömeke K, Liao Y, Gotthardt M, Katus HA, Meder B. Clinical genetics and outcome of left ventricular non-compaction cardiomyopathy. Eur Heart J. 2017;38:3449–60.
77. Fiorillo C, Astrea G, Savarese M, Cassandrini D, Brisca G, Trucco F, Pedemonte M, Trovato R, Ruggiero L, Vercelli L, D'Amico A, Tasca G, Pane M, Fanin M, Bello L, Broda P, Musumeci O, Rodolico C, Messina S, Vita GL, Sframeli M, Gibertini S, Morandi L, Mora M, Maggi L, Petrucci A, Massa R, Grandis M, Toscano A, Pegoraro E, Mercuri E, Bertini E, Mongini T, Santoro L, Nigro V, Minetti C, Santorelli FM, Bruno C, Italian Network on Congenital Myopathies. MYH7-related myopathies: clinical, histopathological and imaging findings in a cohort of Italian patients. Orphanet J Rare Dis. 2016;11:91. https://doi.org/10.1186/s13023-016-0476-1.
78. Tian T, Wang J, Wang H, Sun K, Wang Y, Jia L, Zou Y, Hui R, Zhou X, Song L. A low prevalence of sarcomeric gene variants in a Chinese cohort with left ventricular non-compaction. Heart Vessel. 2015;30:258–64.
79. Finsterer J, Rudnik-Schöneborn S. Myotonic dystrophies: clinical presentation, pathogenesis, diagnostics and therapy. Fortschr Neurol Psychiatr. 2015;83:9–17.
80. Münch G, Bölck B, Sugaru A, Brixius K, Bloch W, Schwinger RH. Increased expression of isoform 1 of the sarcoplasmic reticulum Ca(2+)-release channel in failing human heart. Circulation. 2001;103:2739–44.
81. Finsterer J, Ramaciotti C, Wang CH, Wahbi K, Rosenthal D, Duboc D, Melacini P. Cardiac findings in congenital muscular dystrophies. Pediatrics. 2010;126:538–45.
82. Stöllberger C, Blazek G, Gessner M, Bichler K, Wegner C, Finsterer J. Age-dependency of cardiac and neuromuscular findings in adults with left ventricular hypertrabeculation/noncompaction. Am J Cardiol. 2015;115:1287–92.

Congenital Heart Disease and Noncompaction Cardiomyopathy

4

Annemien E. van den Bosch

Introduction

Although noncompaction cardiomyopathy (NCCM) often occurs in an isolated feature, it may also be present in various types of congenital heart disease (CHD) [1]. In the majority of patients, NCCM is diagnosed in adulthood, similar to hypertrophic cardiomyopathy (HCM) and dilated cardiomyopathy (DCM), which are rarely congenital [2]. In some cases, NCCM detected in adult patients were already present from birth on, but remained unnoticed until symptoms developed and high-resolution cardiac imaging techniques were applied [3]. Recently, the association of NCCM with other cardiac abnormalities has been reported. The pathogenetic mechanism(s) of sarcomere defects in cardiomyopathies are not fully understood. It is possible that the pathological myocardial changes in the adult onset sarcomere related cardiomyopathies are caused by a compensatory response to impaired myocyte function resulting from mutations in the sarcomere genes [4]. However, sarcomere gene mutations found in patients with NCCM were similar to mutations in patients with Ebstein anomaly, but there is no clear genotype-fenotype association [5]. This suggests that sarcomere gene mutations may cause both structural congenital heart disease and NCCM. Longitudinal studies of unaffected carriers of pathogenic mutations are necessary to provide insight whether noncompaction may develop later in life.

A. E. van den Bosch (⊠)
Department of Cardiology, Erasmus MC University Medical Center,
Rotterdam, The Netherlands
e-mail: a.e.vandenbosch@erasmusmc.nl

© Springer Nature Switzerland AG 2019   61
K. Caliskan et al. (eds.), *Noncompaction Cardiomyopathy*,
https://doi.org/10.1007/978-3-030-17720-1_4

Prevalence

With a prevalence of approximately 0.14%, NCCM is a relatively common genetic cardiomyopathy [6]. Although, the original diagnosis of NCCM could only be made in the absence of other structural heart disease, the association of NCCM with other diseases as metabolic diseases, genetic disorders are often reported. Moreover, NCCM is associated with congenital heart disease [7]. Stähli et al. reported the association between NCCM and various forms of congenital malformations [6]. The prevalence of NCCM in patients with CHD differs between the congenital malformations. The most common CHD associated with NCCM were various forms of Ebstein anomaly (15%), aortic coarctation (3%), Tetralogy of Fallot (2%) and bicuspid aortic valve (1%) [6]. In Fig. 4.1, the distribution of NCCM in patients with CHD is shown. Increasingly, congenital cardiac malformations as septal defects, Ebstein anomaly, patent ductus arteriosus, Fallot's tetralogy, aortic coarctation, and aortic aneurysms are being reported in familial cardiomyopathies (HCM, DCM, and NCCM) linked to sarcomere mutations, suggesting that these specific sarcomere defects may have been involved in cardiac morphogenesis. Of note is the congenitally corrected transposition of the great arteries, where the heart twists abnormally during fetal development, and the ventricles are reversed. The heavily trabeculated right ventricle in the left ventricularposition could be confused for a NCCM, a good example of pseudo-NCCM (see Fig. 4.2).

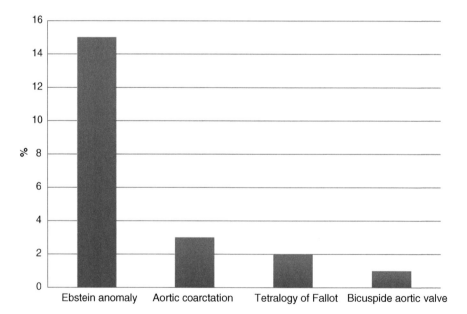

Fig. 4.1 The most common congenital heart disease associated with NCCM

Fig. 4.2 Image of a patient with congenital corrected Transposition of the Great Arteries (ccTGA). The heavily trabeculation of the right ventricle can easily be confused for NCCM

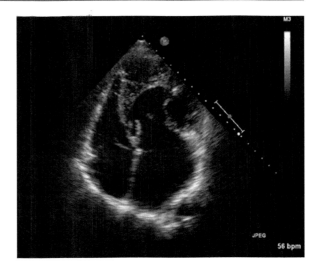

Ebstein Anomaly Associated with Left Ventricular Noncompaction

The most prevalent congenital heart disease associated with left ventricular noncompaction cardiomyopathy is Ebstein anomaly [6]. In the past decade, several reports of Ebstein anomaly associated with noncompaction cardiomyopathy have been described [7–10]. Ebstein anomaly is a rare type of congenital heart disease and has an incidence of approximately 1 in 200,000 live births [9]. Ebstein anomaly is a malformation of the tricuspid valve defined the displacement of the origin of the tricuspid leaflets more apically and rotated to the right ventricular outflow tract. This displacement is accompanied by varying degrees of valvar dysplasia and abnormal attachments, which leads to atrialization of part of the right ventricle with diminished right ventricular size and function. The tricuspid valve itself is usually regurgitant, but may be also stenotic or even imperforate. Transthoracic echocardiography is the main diagnostic modality to confirm the diagnosis of Ebstein anomaly (Figs. 4.3 and 4.4). Late complication as cyanosis, right-sided heart failure, arrhythmias, and sudden cardiac death are reported, although many patients may remain asymptomatic [9]. Therefore, regular cardiologic evaluation is warranted to diagnose early signs of right-heart failure, progressive cardiomegaly with RV dilation, or RV dysfunction. Additionally, rhythm abnormalities as (concealed) accessory pathways, which can lead to Wolff–Parkinson White syndrome are described and other congenital malformation such as atrial septal defect, ventricular septal defect, bicuspid aortic valve or pulmonary stenosis, may also be present. Chronic symptoms in Ebstein anomaly are mainly related to right heart morphology and function. When a patients with Ebstein anomaly and NCCM, the non-compacted myocardium may alter a patient's prognosis because of the high likelihood of ventricular arrhythmia or cardiac arrest [11]. The etiology of Ebstein anomaly is

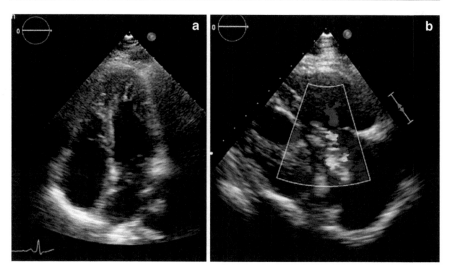

Fig. 4.3 Images of a 32-year-old woman with Ebstein anomaly and left ventricular noncompaction cardiomyopathy. She is asymptomatic and identified as a mutation carrier of MYH7-mutation by family screening. (**a**) Echocardiographic images, apical 4-chamber view; Ebstein anomaly and LVNC are evident. (**b**) Color Doppler image, showing tricuspid valve regurgitation

Fig. 4.4 MRI image, 4-chamber view; Ebstein anomaly is present (shown by apical displacement of the septal leaflet of the tricuspid valve from the insertion of the anterior leaflet of the mitral valve), as well as LVNC. *LV* left atrium, *LA* left atrium, *RV* right ventricle, *RA* right atrium

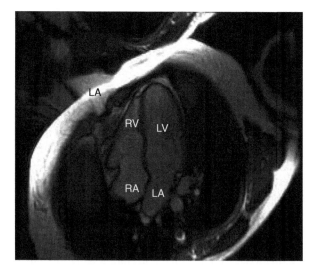

unknown, but families with Ebstein anomaly have been described. The association of Ebstein anomaly and NCCM has been reported similar sarcomeric gene mutations have been found [5]. This suggests that a similar genetic predisposition may lead to both, defective right and left ventricular myocardial differentiation with different morphologic–phenotypic manifestations. Comparable mechanisms may play a role in patients with conotruncal defects in whom the outflow tract of both, the right and left ventricles, and thus differentiation of right and left ventricular myocardial mass may be abnormal. Many reports of NCCM in combination with Ebstein anomaly might describe a specific subtype of Ebstein anomaly, which has an inheritance pattern. Mutations in MYH7 have been reported in sporadic patients as well as families with NCCM and Ebstein anomaly [4]. Therefor, careful screening of patients with Ebstein anomaly for NCCM is preferable. In these patients with confirmed NCCM, further familial and genetic screening are needed with an extra attention for eventual concomitant cardiomyopathy.

Left Ventricular Outflow Tract Abnormalities in Combination with NCCM

Bicuspid aortic valve (BAV) is the most common congenital cardiac malformation, occurring in 1–2% of the general population [12, 13]. BAV is often associated with other common congenital malformations as patent ductus arteriosus, ventricular septal defect, and aortic arch obstruction. However BAV is strongly associated with coarctation of the aorta as well as aortic dilation, aneurysm, and dissection [12, 13]. (Figs. 4.5 and 4.6). Recently, the association of NCCM with less complex CHD, such as LV outflow tract abnormalities, was recognized. Isolated cases of BAV along with NCCM have been described in the literature [14]. Agarwal et al. reported an incidence of up to 11% NCCM in their BAV population [12]. This highlights the need of awareness among clinicians and sonographers aware of the possible presence of NCCM in patients diagnosed with BAV. However, the true incidence of this combination is unknown, and future large-scale studies are needed to understand its true incidence and clinical sequelae. It can be expected that BAV patients with concomitant NCCM are at increased risk for cardiac adverse events. Like concomitant

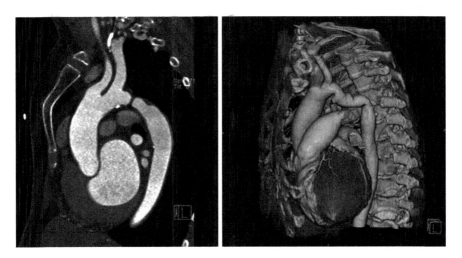

Fig. 4.5 Various forms of aorta coarctation CT images of a patient with aorta coarctation. These images demonstrate the different morphology in aorta coarctation from discrete stenosis to tubular hypoplastic segment, complex 3D turtuous anatomy

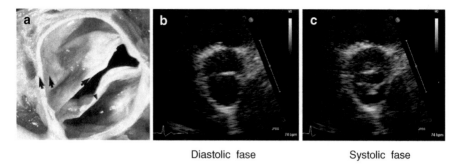

Diastolic fase   Systolic fase

Fig. 4.6 Bicuspid aortic valve (**a**) Anatomic image of a bicuspid aortic valve, (**b** and **c**) Echocardiographic image (parasternal short-axis) from a bicuspid aortic valve in diastole (**b**) and systole (**c**)

aortic valve disease increases the risk for aortic valve stenosis and/or regurgitation and BAV-associated aortopathy for aortic root dissection, concomitant NCCM will increase the risk for heart failure, atrial and ventricular arrhythmias, thromboembolic events, and sudden cardiac death.

Clinical Features

Diagnosis of NCCM relies on non-invasive imaging studies, usually echocardiography and MRI. Transthoracic echocardiography remains the most common diagnostic strategy, largely because of its widespread availability, ease of interpretability, and low cost. The most common diagnostic method is based on a ratio of the thickness of the non-compacted layer to that of the compacted layer, with a ratio of greater than 2:1 at the end of diastole deemed diagnostic as in details described in Chap. 3 [15]. Advanced echocardiographic techniques, such as strain, strain rate, and torsion, are now being used to assist diagnosis of NCCM [16]. In patients with CHD, echocardiography is the first choice for diagnosis and follow-up. However, the awareness to look for NCCM in patients with CHD is not daily practice. Cardiac MRI is now increasingly used in patients with CHD; this might help additionally in identifying additional lesions as NCCM. The MRI diagnostic criteria for NCCM are also based on the ratio of the thickness of the non-compacted layer to that of the compacted layer, with a ratio of greater than > 2.3, given the typically used measurements at the end of diastole [17].

Heart failure is among the most frequent presentations of NCCM, followed by supraventricular and ventricular arrhythmias, including sudden cardiac death, and thrombo-embolic events. However, as in other cardiomyopathies, there is a great variability in clinical presentation, even within families, ranging from a fully asymptomatic course to severe heart failure necessitating cardiac transplantation. Patients with CHD are often diagnosed at childhood and follow for many years. Because the age of presentation of NCCM is highly variable varying, medical and surgical teams caring for patients with CHD should be aware that NCCM can be associated with all forms of CHD and may be associated with poor postoperative outcomes and prolonged lengths of hospital stay [14, 18]. Therefore, patients with NCCM-CHD represent a high-risk population that requires additional attention at the time of preoperative screening, parental counseling and prophylactic drug treatment. Further prospective studies should be performed to further delineate the increased risk associated CHD surgery in children with NCCM.

Therapy and Follow-Up

Current guidelines for heart failure, arrhythmias, cardiac resynchronization therapy, and ICD implantation for primary and secondary prevention are applied for NCCM. For a detailed overview, we refer to the Chaps. 5, 6, and 9. However, the patients with CHD or NCCM have not been included in the landmark trials of ICDs. Also, the patients with CHD face a lot of challenges, because of the multiple previous surgical interventions to address the anatomic malformations, followed by the potential of heart failure and life-threatening arrhythmias. In the study of Gleva, they found that the in-hospital complication rate of ICD procedures in patients with CHD and patients with NCCM were low. However, the CHD patients with Ebstein anomaly, had the greatest all-cause complication rate. In patients with NCCM, beta-blockers and angiotensin-converting enzyme (ACE) – inhibitors are the cornerstones of the treatment in the presence of LV dysfunction and/or arrhythmias. However, clear-cut evidence-based clinical guidelines for this disorder, with or without CHD, are missing due to the lack of data and clinical trials.

An important issue is the use of prophylactic anticoagulants, in view of frequent thrombo-embolic events in NCCM. The early case reports and case series emphasized the high risk of thrombo-embolism and advised routine anticoagulation therapy. However, a review of 22 publications addressing the issue concluded that thromboembolic events are rare in NCCM. Fazio et al. came to the same conclusion. Currently, anticoagulation therapy is advised only in patients with an ejection fraction less than 40% (cut off empirical/arbitrary), paroxysmal or persistent atrial fibrillation, and/or previous thrombo-embolic events. The cardiologic follow-up depends on individual symptoms and cardiac abnormalities. In asymptomatic patients with preserved LV function, annual or biannual cardiologic follow-up is recommended, including ECG and echocardiography. If necessary, these could be extended with 24 h-Holter monitoring and exercise-testing for eventual spontaneous or exercise-induced (non)sustained ventricular tachyarrhythmias.

Conclusion

Various forms of congenital heart disease are associated with NCCM, particularly Ebstein anomaly, left ventricular outflow tract obstruction and tetralogy of Fallot. Medical and surgical teams caring for patients with CHD should be aware that NCCM can be associated with all forms of CHD and may be associated with poor outcomes and increased cardiac events. Further prospective studies should be performed to further delineate the increased risk of patients with CHD in association with NCCM and appropriate management.

Conflict of Interest   None declared.

References

1. Ergul Y, Nisli K, Demirel A, et al. Left ventricular non-compaction in children and adolescents: clinical features, treatment and follow-up. Cardiol J. 2011;18:176–84.
2. Jenni R, Goebel N, Tartini R, Schneider J, Arbenz U, Oelz O. Persisting myocardial sinusoids of both ventricles as an isolated anomaly: echocardiographic, angiographic, and pathologic anatomical findings. Cardiovasc Intervent Radiol. 1986;9:127–31.
3. Engberding R, Bender F. Identification of a rare congenital anomaly of the myocardium by two-dimensional echocardiography: persistence of isolated myocardial sinusoids. Am J Cardiol. 1984;53:1733–4.
4. Postma AV, van Engelen K, van de Meerakker J, et al. Mutations in the sarcomere gene MYH7 in Ebstein anomaly. Circ Cardiovasc Genet. 2011;4:43–50.
5. Klaassen S, Probst S, Oechslin E, et al. Mutations in sarcomere protein genes in left ventricular noncompaction. Circulation. 2008;117:2893–901.
6. Stähli BE, Gebhard C, Biaggi P, Klaassen S, Valsangiacomo Buechel E, Attenhofer Jost CH, et al. Left ventricular non-compaction: prevalence in congenital heart disease. Int J Cardiol. 2013;167:2477–81.
7. Aras D, Tufekcioglu O, Ergun K, et al. Clinical features of isolated ventricular noncompaction in adults long-term clinical course, echocardiographic properties, and predictors of left ventricular failure. J Card Fail. 2006;12:726–33.
8. Attenhofer Jost CH, Connolly HM, Warnes CA, et al. Noncompacted myocardium in Ebstein's anomaly: initial description in three patients. J Am Soc Echocardiogr. 2004;17:677–80.
9. Attenhofer Jost CH, Connolly HM, Dearani JA, Edwards WD, Danielson GK. Ebstein's anomaly. Circulation. 2007;115:277–85.
10. Pignatelli RH, Texter KM, Denfield SW, Grenier MA, Altman CA, Ayres NA, et al. LV noncompaction in Ebstein's anomaly in infants and outcomes. JACC Cardiovasc Imaging. 2014;7:207–9.
11. Attenhofer Jost CH, Connolly HM, O'Leary PW, Warnes CA, Tajik AJ, Seward JB. Left heart lesions in patients with Ebstein anomaly. Mayo Clin Proc. 2005;80:361–8.
12. Agarwal A, Khandheria BK, et al. Left ventricular noncompaction in patients with bicuspid aortic valve. JASE. 2013;26(11):1306–13.
13. Fedak PW, Verma S, David TE, Leask RL, Weisel RD, Butany J. Clinical and pathophysiological implications of a bicuspid aortic valve. Circulation. 2002;106:900–4.
14. Cavusoglu Y, Ata N, Timuralp B, Gorenek B, Goktekin O, Kudaiberdieva G, et al. Noncompaction of the ventricular myocardium: report of two cases with bicuspid aortic valve demonstrating poor prognosis and with prominent right ventricular involvement. Echocardiography. 2003;20:379–83.
15. Lang RM, Bierig M, Devereux RB, Flachskampf FA, Foster E, Pellikka PA, et al. Recommendations for chamber quantification: a report from the American Society of Echocardiography's Guidelines and Standards Committee and the Chamber Quantification Writing Group, developed in conjunction with the European Association of Echocardiography, a branch of the European Society of Cardiology. J Am Soc Echocardiogr. 2005;18:1440–63.
16. van Dalen BM, Caliskan K, Soliman OI, Nemes A, Vletter WB, Ten Cate FJ, et al. Left ventricular solid body rotation in non-compaction cardiomyopathy: a potential new objective and quantitative functional diagnostic criterion? Eur J Heart Fail. 2008;10:1088–93.

17. Petersen SE, Selvanayagam JB, Wiesmann F, Robson MD, Francis JM, Anderson RH, et al. Left ventricular non-compaction: insights from cardiovascular magnetic resonance imaging. J Am Coll Cardiol. 2005;46:101–5.
18. Ohki S, Moriyama Y, Mohara J, Kimura C, Sata N, Miyahara K. Aortic valve replacement for aortic regurgitation in a patient with left ventricular noncompaction. Ann Thorac Surg. 2009;87:290–2.

Malignant Arrhythmias and Sudden Cardiac Death in Patients with Noncompaction Cardiomyopathy: Prevalence, Prevention, and Use of Implantable Cardiac Defibrillators

5

Emrah Kaya, Martijn Otten, Sing-Chien Yap, Tamas Szili-Torok, and Kadir Caliskan

Introduction

Noncompaction cardiomyopathy (NCCM) was first described almost a half century ago, it initially began as an unusual autopsy finding [1, 2]. Over the past three decades increased interest and dedicated research have given us more insight about this relatively uncommon and new clinicopathologic entity. However, questions regarding the appropriate diagnosis, management, and prognosis remain unanswered. NCCM is now recognized as a distinct primary genetic cardiomyopathy by the American Heart Association (AHA) and as unclassified cardiomyopathy by the European Society of Cardiology (ESC) [3, 4]. This cardiomyopathy could have poor prognosis in certain adult patients [5, 6]. In childhood the consequences of this disease can be more severe and is often associated with other congenital anomalies [7]. NCCM has a highly variable clinical presentation and is usually diagnosed when the condition becomes symptomatic or when complications occur in patients. These complications are chronic heart failure, lethal arrhythmias and thromboembolic events [8–10]. But, Sudden cardiac death (SCD) is the most devastation outcome. The mortality in patients with NCCM has been reported in 18% of adults and 0–13% in children [11].

E. Kaya
Thoraxcenter, Department of Cardiology, Erasmus MC University Medical Center, Rotterdam, The Netherlands

Department of Cardiology, Onze Lieve Vrouwe Gasthuis, Amsterdam, The Netherlands

M. Otten · S.-C. Yap · T. Szili-Torok
Thoraxcenter, Department of Cardiology, Erasmus MC University Medical Center, Rotterdam, The Netherlands

K. Caliskan (✉)
Erasmus MC University Medical Center, Department of Cardiology, Rotterdam, The Netherlands
e-mail: k.caliskan@erasmusmc.nl

© Springer Nature Switzerland AG 2019
K. Caliskan et al. (eds.), *Noncompaction Cardiomyopathy*,
https://doi.org/10.1007/978-3-030-17720-1_5

SCD is defined as death from cardiac causes with an abrupt loss of conscious-ness less than 1 h after the onset of the symptoms. In the usual clinical practice, coronary artery disease is often the culprit of sudden cardiac death, approximately 65–70%; and with almost 10% of deaths in patients with non-ischemic cardiomy-opathies [12]. Non-ischemic cardiomyopathies include hypertrophic cardiomy-opathy, dilated cardiomyopathy, arrhythmogenic right ventricular cardiomyopathy, takotsubo cardiomyopathy, cardiac amyloidosis, cardiac sarcoidosis and also NCCM. Most sudden cardiac deaths within the NCCM population are due to malignant ventricular arrhythmias, specifically caused by ventricular tachycardia (VT), ventricular fibrillation (VF), with some due to asystole [13, 14]. As an unex-pected event, it has devastating effect for the patients and families.

The implantable cardioverter defibrillator (ICD) is the single most effective therapy to prevent sudden death in patients resuscitated from sudden cardiac arrest or after an episode of sustained VT [15]. In patients with ischemic heart disease several large, randomized, multicenter trials have shown the superiority of the ICD over drug (anti-arrhythmic) therapy for both primary and secondary pre-vention of sudden death [16, 17]. Studies about the role of ICD's in the prevention of SCD however, are limited in NCCM patients [18]. Furthurmore, the application of ICD therapy in relatively young patients with NCCM for primary prevention has only recently become a focus [19]. Although there is a general consensus that NCCM patients who survive cardiac arrest with VF should be offered ICD for secondary prevention, those patients represent a small portion of the at-risk population.

Epidemiological Overview

In the general population, NCCM is reported in infants at a frequency of 0.80 per 100,000 individuals per year, in children, the incidence is found to be 0.12 per 100,000 individuals per year and in adults 0.05% [6, 23, 30]. In patients with heart failure, the prevalence of NCCM was up to 3-4% [22, 23]. Age at which NCCM is recognized is highly variable, ranging from early infancy to late adult-hood [24]. The true prevalence of NCCM may be even higher, because asymp-tomatic individuals may go unnoticed in studies. Due to increased awareness of NCCM, as wel as the improvement of modern imaging modalities, including cardiac magnetic resonance imaging and CT-scan, the incidence of NCCM will probably increase in the future. Albeith SCD is the most striking complication of NCCM, it is usually believed to occur in relatively small percentage of the population. A large pediatric study in NCCM reports the risk of sudden death to be 6% [20]. However, recent studies have shown sudden death ranging from 13 to 18% in adults and 0–13% in the children with NCCM [11]. The children who did poorly often showed rhythm abnormalities related to sudden death as a pre-dominant sign [20]. The variable prevalence of SCD can be probably best explained by the diagnostic criteria applied for NCCM, length of follow-up and the studied population [6, 20–26]. There is currently no consensus on absolute diagnostic criteria, which limits the strength of the conclusion regarding exact prevalence and incidence of sudden death in NCCM. Furthermore, epidemiological research in NCCM is often based on retrospective studies of patients referred for echocardiography [10, 27, 28].

A variety of arrhythmias has been identified in association with NCCM, including bundle branch reentry, idiopathic VT, right ventricular outflow tract (RVOT) origin, left bundle branch and right bundle branch morphologies, bidirectional, fascicular VT, polymorphic and VF [27–32]. But malignant ventricular tachyarrhythmia's (VA's), including cardiac arrest due to VT/VF, have been considered as the hallmark [29]. Ventricular arrhythmias are reported in 38–47% in adult NCCM population and 0–38% in children with NCCM [11, 22]. In our series, 14 out of 84 patients (16.7%) presented primarily with SCD/VA's [34].

Pathophysiology of SCD/VA in the NCCM population

Substantial data from several electrocardiograms and Holter's show that sudden death events in NCCM are caused by sustained ventricular tachyarrhythmias, like rapid ventricular tachycardia (VT) and/or ventricular fibrillation [13, 44, 45].

However, the pathogenesis of arrhythmia's in NCCM patients is still poorly understood. It has been hypothesized that an arrest in the embryogenic development of the heart, results in disturbed compaction process of the myocardium. Normal myocardium gradually compacts from the epicardium inward and capillaries are formed by the compressed intertrabecular recesses [8]. Concurrent inappropriate maturation of the primary cardiac conduction system could cause a more pronounced manifestation of rhythm disturbances [21, 47, 51]. Histological examination shows myocardium around deep intertrabecular recesses that may serve as slow conducting zones with reentry. Impaired flow reserve, causing intermittent ischemia, may play a role [51]. Subendocardial ischemia and coronary microcirculation disturbances could cause VT and VF [47]. It has been also hypothesized that abnormalities of the cardiac conduction system or intramyocardial fibrosis and scar formation could be a trigger. Recently, we described a mismatch between the origin of premature ventricular complexes (PVC's) and the noncompacted segments in NCCM. The PVC's on the surface electrocardiograms of NCCM patients looked mainly originating from the conduction system and related myocardium [41]. In another case series of 9 patients by Muser et al. VA substrate typically localized in the mid-apical LV segments, whereas focal PVCs often arisen from LV basal–septal regions and/or papillary muscles [42]. In a case report by Casella et al., electroanatomic mapping in a 43-year old man, ventricular noncompaction is characterized by electrical abnormalities including low voltage and scar areas, mainly related to the presence and extent of myocardial fibrosis rather than noncompacted myocardium [43].

According to current guidelines frequent PVCs and runs of NSVT in subjects with a prior myocardial infarction have been associated with an increased risk of death [52]. In contrast, in patients with non-ischemic cardiomyopathy, PVCs do not appear to be associated with a worse prognosis although data are limited [53]. In a recent study no statistically significant correlation could be found between the origin of PVCs and the occurrence of a previous spontaneous VT. Also the data suggest that PVCs in NCCM originate mainly from areas that are not affected echocardiographically by NCCM [54].

Also, prior theories about ventricular arrhythmias in NCCM involve microreentry in the trabeculated myocardium, epicardial coronary hypoperfusion, and concurrent developmental arrest of the conduction system [55]. However, electrophysiological mapping in NCCM patients with sustained VT did not reveal the anatomical substrate. Another relevant finding in recent years, is a high prevalence of early repolarization (ER) being reported in patients presenting with cardiac arrest or sudden cardiac death (Fig. 5.1). Previous studies showed a high prevalence of ER in NCCM patients, especially in those patients presenting with malignant ventricular arrhythmias (75%). Interestingly, early repolarization was also frequently observed (31%) in NCCM patients not presenting with ventricular arrhythmias [13, 29].

The pathophysiology of ER and associated arrhythmias in NCCM remains unclear. Increased regional trabeculation, with deep intramyocardial invaginations carrying the Purkinje system deeper into the mid-myocardium, as in NCCM, may cause inhomogeneous depolarization and repolarization. This transmural heterogeneity may result in the development of (malignant) ventricular arrhythmias [29]. This looks be in line with the recent findings that show, that normal LV twist is absent in patients with

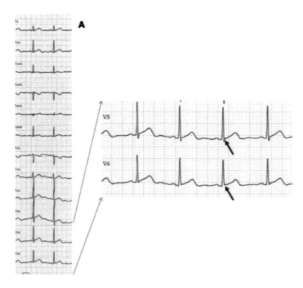

Fig. 5.1 Leads V5–V6 On the surface electrocardiogram of a patient with noncompaction cardiomyopahty who survived a sudden cardiac arrest due to ventricular fibrillation (VF): there were early repolarization both in inferior and lateral leads (arrows only for leads V5–V6 are shown)

NCCM, which is probably due to also an immature endocardial helical system. Further studies are needed to identify the mechanism of the arrhythmias in NCCM to adopt an appropriate therapeutic approach for this distinct patient group.

Case Report

A 35-year old woman was admitted to the cardiology department because of palpitations. A 24-h Holter monitor and an echocardiogram were ordered after routine control. The 24h-Holter showed frequent PVCs and nonsustained VTs (Fig. 5.2a, b) and

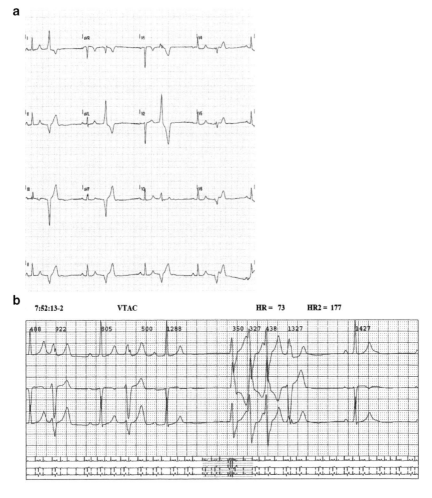

Fig. 5.2 (**a**) Electrocardiogram showing frequent premature ventricular beats in a patient with NCCM. (**b**) Holter study showing multiple PVC's and a bradycardia-related nonsustained VT in patient with NCCM

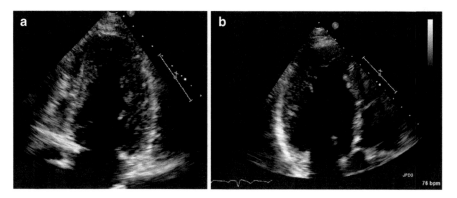

Fig. 5.3 (**a**) Four-chamber view of this patient demonstrating extensive trabeculation in the apical and lateral LV walls. (**b**) three chamber view, showing extensive trabeculation in posterior wall

the echocardiogram showed characteristics of "asymmetrical hypertrophic cardio-myopathy". The patient received ACE inhibitors, she didn't continue the beta-blockers, probably because of intolerance. After her discharge from the hospital, the patient remained a couple years asymptomatic. Unfortunately, 3 years after the initial presentation, she was again admitted but now because of an out-of-hospital cardiac arrest. She had collapsed suddenly in a grocery store and was resuscitated by bystand-ers. Ambulance had arrived after 6 min and the ECG monitor showed ventricular fibrillation. She was successfully resuscitated. During her hospitalization a new echocardiogram revealed moderate LV dysfunction (LVEF 35%) and heavy trabecu-lations were noted at the posterior and apical walls (Fig. 5.3a, b). Considering the NCCM with decreased LVEF and VF as complication, an ICD device according to current guidelines was successfully implanted for secondary prophylaxes. The patient received drug therapy and she was discharged without complications. After the implantation of the ICD, she had several appropriate ICD shocks with need of adjustment of the medical therapy (Fig. 5.3). Last years, the patient remains stable, NYHA class I, with also stable moderate LV dysfunction.

Clinical Presentation

NCCM is a heterogeneous and unforeseeable disease with respect to its natural his-tory and clinical expression. A significant number of affected individuals go unrec-ognized or only have intermittent symptoms. The symptomatic NCCM patients may have (atypical) chest pain, dyspnea (with or without exertion), palpitations, edema, syncope, embolic ischemic stroke, myocardial infarction, pulmonary embolism, or sudden cardiac death [10]. Patients, whether adults or pediatric, should undergo a careful history taking and physical examination, with specific attention to cardiac symptoms such as unexplained syncope, palpitations and discomfort on the chest. Also, a thorough family history of CMPs and SCD should be obtained. Major clinical manifestations of NCCM are: heart failure, supraventricular of ventricular arrhythmias, and/or thrombo-embolic events [40]. In this chapter we will focus on the presentation, diagnosis and managment of malignant ventricular arrhythmias and sudden cardiac death.

Patients with NCCM are often accompanied by electrocardiographic abnormalities. The frequency of these abnormalities is high, approximately 90% in adults and in pediatric patients [11]. However, these ECG findings were thought to be not specific [56]. Although, conduction delay and QTc prolongation were correlated with reduced systolic function and LV hypertrophy was significantly associated with thromboembolism. Against that, patients with normal ECGs at presentation had often a preserved left ventricular ejection fractions (LVEF) [29].

Supraventricular arrhythmias and conduction abnormalities are relatively common in NCCM patients. They occur in up to one-quarter of the patients, including atrial fibrillation, atrial flutter, paroxysmal supraventricular tachycardia, or complete atrioventricular block [21–23]. The symptoms may manifest as palpitations, (near) syncope or heart failure, with potiential tachycardiomyopathy. Atrial fibrillation occurs in 5–29% of adult patients with NCCM but has not been described in pediatric patients. Wolff-Parkinson-White syndrome found often in patients with NCCM [11]. Wolff-Parkinson-White syndrome is one of the best known preexcitation syndromes. It is characterized by the presence of an accessory pathway which predisposes tachyarrhythmias and sudden death. Wolff-Parkinson-White syndrome was found often in pediatric patients 13–15% and in 0–3% of adult patients with NCCM [11, 57, 58] . Also, sinus node dysfunction can be a clinical manifestation of NCCM. Recently, association with ion channel gene HCN4 mutation is described linked to sinus bradycardia and NCCM.

Ventricular arrhythmias are since its initial description prevalent in patients with NCCM in both adults as in children. In a study of 17 adult patients with NCCM, VT was observed in almost the half of the patients during a follow-up of 30 months. Five out of these 8 patients died during the follow up. An impaired left ventricular systolic function was seen in 82% of the patients [23]. Electric instability can lead to short episodes of VT, also termed as non-sustained VT. If sustained, it can be life threatening and could lead to hemodynamic compromise. Between VT in NCCM and impaired systolic function there seems to be a correlation, but it can't be concluded that a normal systolic function excludes the risk of VT [13]. In our study, about the indications for an implantable cardioverter defibrillator therapy and the outcomes in 77 adult NCCM patients, 44 of them had such a device according to the guidelines for non-ischaemic cardiomyopathy. During a follow-up (mean) of 33 months, eight patients presented with appropriate defibrillator shocks as a result of sustained ventricular tachycardia. Most of patients implanted with an ICD for secondary prophylaxis has minimal LV dysfunction and no HF. This suggests that patients with NCCM could be at high risk for sudden cardiac death regardless of the presence of HF and/or significant LV dysfunction [19].

Diagnosis and Risk Stratification

Early diagnosis of noncompaction cardiomyopathy can be challenging, given the low prevalence in general practice [23, 25, 60]. Another important factor is the phenotypic heterogeneity of the population [29, 61]. Clinical presentation can be variable from asymptomatic patients to end-stage heart failure, or supraventricular, ventricular arrhythmias, including ventricular tachycardia, ventricular fibrillation and sudden cardiac death. Moreover, no consensus has been reached yet regarding the diagnostic criteria and the best diagnostic approach. Therefore, pathomorphological findings currently appear to be the gold standard for diagnosing NCCM with Jenni criteria most useful for the daily clinical practice [27]. The debate on the true incidence and prevalence of malignant ventricular arrhythmias in NCCM patients continues, because of the lack of large-scale controlled, randomized trials. Thus, definitive risk factors for SCD remains speculative.

The annual incidence of SCD in the general population is 0.1–0.2%, specific subgroups of patients like coronary artery disease and reduced LV function, dilated cardiomyopathy (DCM), arrhytmogenic cardiomyopathy (ARVC), hypertrophic cardiomyopathy (HCM), Brugada syndrome, long QT syndrome, and NCCM are at higher risk. The only way for appropriate risk stratification is by collecting relevant clinical data in a multi-center, prospective registry and follow-up studies. This is however lacking in most nonischemic cardiomyopathies, with no exception for the new disease entity of NCCM. Despite lack of definitive risk factors, it is still important to evaluate each patient for potential risk factors for SCD. The risk factors for SCD that are most commonly cited include: increased LV size, decreased LV systolic function, and the presence of ventricular arrhythmias [6, 20, 25]. Possible other high-risk features are symptomatic heart failure (NYHA class: II to IV) and atrial fibrillation in adults and repolarization abnormalities (ST changes and T wave inversion) in pediatric patients may also indicate a poor outcome [26, 29]. Therefore, periodic echocardiogram and Holter recordings are recommended [20]. Risk of SCD seems greatest in pediatric patients, less than 1 year of age [6, 20, 25]. Subsequent studies showed that sex, localization, and degree of (non)compaction did not seem to be risk factors. Inducible arrhythmias during electrophysiology (EP) testing has been suggested to be useful in NCCM, however it has not been shown to be a reliable predictor of SCD in NCCM patients. But, it must be said that data regarding EP is limited. The usefulness of EP for risk stratification in NCCM remains to be determined [9]. In the following section, we describe out current clinical approach in the view of the scarce contemporary evidence, but with a our more than decade experience with a broad spectrum of NCCM patients.

Management

ICD therapy is an effective therapy to prevent sudden cardiac death. The ICD therapy can be applied for primary and secondary prevention. Primary prevention means that individuals are at high risk for, but did not yet have an episode of sustained VT,

VF or resuscitated cardiac arrest, especially in the presence of spontaneous ventricular unrest in the form of frequent premature ventricular complexes and/or nonsustained VT. ICD therapy is applied for secondary prevention in patients who have been resuscitated from cardiac arrest or present with documented, sustained ventricular tachyarrhythmia, or unexplained (near)-syncope. Current guidelines recommend implantation of an ICD in patients with impaired left ventricular (LV) function (LVEF ≤35%) caused by coronary artery disease or cardiomyopathy [15, 63]. Ventricular tachyarrhytmias, including cardiac arrest due to VT/VF, are reported in 38–47% and sudden death in 13–18% of adult patients with NCCM [6, 64]. Therefore, implantation of an ICD in these patients is a valid option, although in previous trials no known NCCM patients were included. However, no specific risk factors for SCD in NCCM patients have yet been identified [13]. In our center, our approach for risk stratification of SCD in NCCM patients, whether symptomatic or asymptomatic, is described in the flowchart, (Fig. 5.4). For secondary prevention of sudden cardiac death, an ICD is always advised. If there is a significant dysfunction (i.e. LVEF ≤35%), especially in the setting of symptoms or signs of systolic heart failure, a prophylactic ICD for primary prevention is advised. In other patients empiric individualized risk stratification should be applied, after through anamnesis, physical examination, ECG, an exercise test, and a 48h-Holter. If spontaneous ventricular unrest is found, i.e. nonsustained VT's, especially in the setting of systolic LV dysfunction (LVEF <50%), familial history of premature SCD <50 years, early repolarization and/or fragmented QRS on the 12-leads ECG, a prophylactic

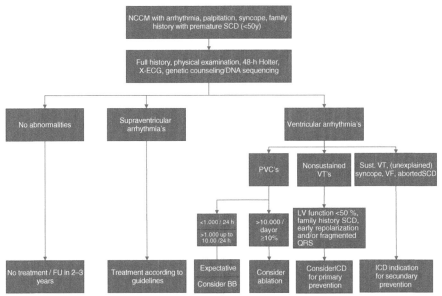

SCD sudden cardiac death; PVC premature ventricularcontraction; VT ventriculartachycardia; VF ventricularfibrilation; BB beta-blocker

Fig. 5.4 Flowchart for the risk stratification for sudden cardiac death and management of NCCM patients

ICD should be considered after through extensive counseling and shared-decision making. With this empiric approach, no episode of SCD, sustained VT or syncope had been encountered in our national referral center for NCCM in the Netherlands with > 200 outpatient patients and up to 15 years of follow-up.

Information on the long-term outcome after ICD therapy in this population remains however limited. Caliskan et al. investigated the indications and outcomes of ICDs in 77 adult patients with NCCM, of whom 44 had a device implanted on the basis of current guidelines for non-ischaemic cardiomyopathy. During a mean follow up of 34 months, eight patients presented with appropriate ICD shocks because of sustained VT after a median of 6 months. The relatively high percentage of appropriate shocks for sustained VT in our population confirms that these NCCM patients are at high risk for SCD and that implanting ICD in this population is an appropriate approach.

It is an interesting finding to see that all the appropriate ICD interventions in our population were due to (fast) VTs, although it isn't known whether the initial rhythm from our SCD/VF patients was also started with a VT.

Conclusion

In conclusion, in patients with NCCM, malignant ventricular arrhythmia's and sudden cardiac death are frequently encountered. In selected patients, an ICD implantation in these patients is a valid option and highly effective. Until we have reliable prospective data, it remains reasonable to use the current guidelines for management of patients with VA and the prevention of SCD in non-ischemic cardiomyopathy patients.

References

1. Feldt RH, Rahimtoola SH, Davis GD, Swan HJ, Titus JL. Anomalous ventricular myocardial patterns in a child with complex congenital heart disease. Am J Cardiol. 1969;23:732–4.
2. Finsterer J, Zarrouk-Mahjoub S. Grant et al. 1926 did not provide the first description of left ventricular hypertrabeculation/noncompaction. Int J Cardiol. 2013;169:e51–2.
3. Maron BJ, Towbin JA, Thiene G, Antzelevitch C, Corrado D, Arnett D, Moss AJ, Seidman CE, Young JB, American Heart Association, Council on Clinical Cardiology, Heart Failure and Transplantation Committee, Quality of Care and Outcomes Research and Functional Genomics and Translational Biology Interdisciplinary Working Groups, Council on Epidemiology and Prevention. Contemporary definitions and classification of the cardiomyopathies: an American Heart Association scientific statement from the council on clinical cardiology, heart failure and transplantation committee; quality of care and outcomes research and functional genomics and translational biology interdisciplinary working groups; and council on epidemiology and prevention. Circulation. 2006;113:1807–16.
4. Elliott P, Andersson B, Arbustini E, Bilinska Z, Cecchi F, Charron P, Dubourg O, Kuhl U, Maisch B, McKenna WJ, Monserrat L, Pankuweit S, Rapezzi C, Seferovic P, Tavazzi L, Keren A. Classification of the cardiomyopathies: a position statement from the European Society of Cardiology Working Group on Myocardial and Pericardial Diseases. Eur Heart J. 2008;29:270–6.

5. Kobza R, Jenni R, Erne P, Oechslin E, Duru F. Implantable cardioverter-defibrillators in patients with left ventricular noncompaction. Pacing Clin Electrophysiol. 2008;31:461–7.
6. Oechslin EN, Attenhofer Jost CH, Rojas JR, Kaufmann PA, Jenni R. Long-term follow-up of 34 adults with isolated left ventricular noncompaction: a distinct cardiomyopathy with poor prognosis. J Am Coll Cardiol. 2000;36:493–500.
7. Stollberger C, Finsterer J. Unmet needs in the cardiologic and neurologic work-up of left ventricular hypertrabeculation/noncompaction. Expert Rev Cardiovasc Ther. 2016;14:1151–60.
8. Jenni R, Oechslin EN, van der Loo B. Isolated ventricular non-compaction of the myocardium in adults. Heart. 2007;93:11–5.
9. Steffel J, Kobza R, Namdar M, Wolber T, Brunckhorst C, Luscher TF, Jenni R, Duru F. Electrophysiological findings in patients with isolated left ventricular non-compaction. Europace. 2009;11:1193–200.
10. Finsterer J, Stollberger C, Towbin JA. Left ventricular noncompaction cardiomyopathy: cardiac, neuromuscular, and genetic factors. Nat Rev Cardiol. 2017;14:224–37.
11. Weiford BC, Subbarao VD, Mulhern KM. Noncompaction of the ventricular myocardium. Circulation. 2004;109:2965–71.
12. Kannel WB, Thomas HE Jr. Sudden coronary death: the Framingham Study. Ann N Y Acad Sci. 1982;382:3–21.
13. Stollberger C, Finsterer J. Arrhythmias and left ventricular hypertrabeculation /noncompaction. Curr Pharm Des. 2010;16:2880–94.
14. Soni A, LeLorier P. Sudden death in nondilated cardiomyopathies: pathophysiology and prevention. Curr Heart Fail Rep. 2005;2:118–23.
15. Zipes DP, Camm AJ, Borggrefe M, Buxton AE, Chaitman B, Fromer M, Gregoratos G, Klein G, Moss AJ, Myerburg RJ, Priori SG, Quinones MA, Roden DM, Silka MJ, Tracy C, Smith SC Jr, Jacobs AK, Adams CD, Antman EM, Anderson JL, Hunt SA, Halperin JL, Nishimura R, Ornato JP, Page RL, Riegel B, Blanc JJ, Budaj A, Dean V, Deckers JW, Despres C, Dickstein K, Lekakis J, McGregor K, Metra M, Morais J, Osterspey A, Tamargo JL, Zamorano JL, American College of Cardiology/American Heart Association Task Force, European Society of Cardiology Committee for Practice Guidelines, European Heart Rhythm Association and Heart Rhythm Society. ACC/AHA/ESC 2006 guidelines for management of patients with ventricular arrhythmias and the prevention of sudden cardiac death: a report of the American College of Cardiology/American Heart Association Task Force and the European Society of Cardiology Committee for Practice Guidelines (writing committee to develop guidelines for management of patients with ventricular arrhythmias and the prevention of sudden cardiac death): developed in collaboration with the European Heart Rhythm Association and the Heart Rhythm Society. Circulation. 2006;114:e385–484.
16. Antiarrhythmics versus Implantable Defibrillators (AVID) Investigators. A comparison of antiarrhythmic-drug therapy with implantable defibrillators in patients resuscitated from near-fatal ventricular arrhythmias. N Engl J Med. 1997;337:1576–83.
17. Moss AJ, Zareba W, Hall WJ, Klein H, Wilber DJ, Cannom DS, Daubert JP, Higgins SL, Brown MW, Andrews ML, Multicenter Automatic Defibrillator Implantation Trial II Investigators. Prophylactic implantation of a defibrillator in patients with myocardial infarction and reduced ejection fraction. N Engl J Med. 2002;346:877–83.
18. Kobza R, Steffel J, Erne P, Schoenenberger AW, Hurlimann D, Luscher TF, Jenni R, Duru F. Implantable cardioverter-defibrillator and cardiac resynchronization therapy in patients with left ventricular noncompaction. Heart Rhythm. 2010;7:1545–9.
19. Caliskan K, Szili-Torok T, Theuns DA, Kardos A, Geleijnse ML, Balk AH, van Domburg RT, Jordaens L, Simoons ML. Indications and outcome of implantable cardioverter-defibrillators for primary and secondary prophylaxis in patients with noncompaction cardiomyopathy. J Cardiovasc Electrophysiol. 2011;22:898–904.
20. Brescia ST, Rossano JW, Pignatelli R, Jefferies JL, Price JF, Decker JA, Denfield SW, Dreyer WJ, Smith O, Towbin JA, Kim JJ. Mortality and sudden death in pediatric left ventricular noncompaction in a tertiary referral center. Circulation. 2013;127:2202–8.

21. Chin TK, Perloff JK, Williams RG, Jue K, Mohrmann R. Isolated noncompaction of left ventricular myocardium. A study of eight cases. Circulation. 1990;82:507–13.
22. Ichida F, Hamamichi Y, Miyawaki T, Ono Y, Kamiya T, Akagi T, Hamada H, Hirose O, Isobe T, Yamada K, Kurotobi S, Mito H, Miyake T, Murakami Y, Nishi T, Shinohara M, Seguchi M, Tashiro S, Tomimatsu H. Clinical features of isolated noncompaction of the ventricular myocardium: long-term clinical course, hemodynamic properties, and genetic background. J Am Coll Cardiol. 1999;34:233–40.
23. Ritter M, Oechslin E, Sutsch G, Attenhofer C, Schneider J, Jenni R. Isolated noncompaction of the myocardium in adults. Mayo Clin Proc. 1997;72:26–31.
24. Lofiego C, Biagini E, Pasquale F, Ferlito M, Rocchi G, Perugini E, Bacchi-Reggiani L, Boriani G, Leone O, Caliskan K, ten Cate FJ, Picchio FM, Branzi A, Rapezzi C. Wide spectrum of presentation and variable outcomes of isolated left ventricular non-compaction. Heart. 2007;93:65–71.
25. Aras D, Tufekcioglu O, Ergun K, Ozeke O, Yildiz A, Topaloglu S, Deveci B, Sahin O, Kisacik HL, Korkmaz S. Clinical features of isolated ventricular noncompaction in adults long-term clinical course, echocardiographic properties, and predictors of left ventricular failure. J Card Fail. 2006;12:726–33.
26. Stollberger C, Blazek G, Wegner C, Finsterer J. Heart failure, atrial fibrillation and neuromuscular disorders influence mortality in left ventricular hypertrabeculation/noncompaction. Cardiology. 2011;119:176–82.
27. Burke A, Mont E, Kutys R, Virmani R. Left ventricular noncompaction: a pathological study of 14 cases. Hum Pathol. 2005;36:403–11.
28. Hussein A, Karimianpour A, Collier P, Krasuski RA. Isolated noncompaction of the left ventricle in adults. J Am Coll Cardiol. 2015;66:578–85.
29. Miyake CY, Kim JJ. Arrhythmias in left ventricular noncompaction. Card Electrophysiol Clin. 2015;7:319–30.
30. Arbustini E, Weidemann F, Hall JL. Left ventricular noncompaction: a distinct cardiomyopathy or a trait shared by different cardiac diseases? J Am Coll Cardiol. 2014;64:1840–50.
31. Pignatelli RH, McMahon CJ, Dreyer WJ, Denfield SW, Price J, Belmont JW, Craigen WJ, Wu J, El Said H, Bezold LI, Clunie S, Fernbach S, Bowles NE, Towbin JA. Clinical characterization of left ventricular noncompaction in children: a relatively common form of cardiomyopathy. Circulation. 2003;108:2672–8.
32. Nugent AW, Daubeney PE, Chondros P, Carlin JB, Colan SD, Cheung M, Davis AM, Chow CW, Weintraub RG, National Australian Childhood Cardiomyopathy Study. Clinical features and outcomes of childhood hypertrophic cardiomyopathy: results from a national population-based study. Circulation. 2005;112:1332–8.
33. Kovacevic-Preradovic T, Jenni R, Oechslin EN, Noll G, Seifert B, Attenhofer Jost CH. Isolated left ventricular noncompaction as a cause for heart failure and heart transplantation: a single center experience. Cardiology. 2009;112:158–64.
34. Patrianakos AP, Parthenakis FI, Nyktari EG, Vardas PE. Noncompaction myocardium imaging with multiple echocardiographic modalities. Echocardiography. 2008;25:898–900.
35. Goud A, Padmanabhan S. A rare form of cardiomyopathy: left ventricular non-compaction cardiomyopathy. J Community Hosp Intern Med Perspect. 2016;6:29888.
36. Stollberger C, Finsterer J, Blazek G. Left ventricular hypertrabeculation/noncompaction and association with additional cardiac abnormalities and neuromuscular disorders. Am J Cardiol. 2002;90:899–902.
37. Jefferies JL, Wilkinson JD, Sleeper LA, Colan SD, Lu M, Pahl E, Kantor PF, Everitt MD, Webber SA, Kaufman BD, Lamour JM, Canter CE, Hsu DT, Addonizio LJ, Lipshultz SE, Towbin JA, Pediatric Cardiomyopathy Registry Investigators. Cardiomyopathy phenotypes and outcomes for children with left ventricular myocardial noncompaction: results from the pediatric cardiomyopathy registry. J Card Fail. 2015;21:877–84.
38. Kohli SK, Pantazis AA, Shah JS, Adeyemi B, Jackson G, McKenna WJ, Sharma S, Elliott PM. Diagnosis of left-ventricular non-compaction in patients with left-ventricular systolic dysfunction: time for a reappraisal of diagnostic criteria? Eur Heart J. 2008;29:89–95.

39. Peters F, Khandheria BK, dos Santos C, Matioda H, Maharaj N, Libhaber E, Mamdoo F, Essop MR. Isolated left ventricular noncompaction in sub-Saharan Africa: a clinical and echocardiographic perspective. Circ Cardiovasc Imaging. 2012;5:187–93.
40. Towbin JA, Jefferies JL. Cardiomyopathies due to left ventricular noncompaction, mitochondrial and storage diseases, and inborn errors of metabolism. Circ Res. 2017;121:838–54.
41. Lauer RM, Fink HP, Petry EL, Dunn MI, Diehl AM. Angiographic demonstration of intramyocardial sinusoids in pulmonary-valve atresia with intact ventricular septum and hypoplastic right ventricle. N Engl J Med. 1964;271:68–72.
42. Sedmera D, Pexieder T, Vuillemin M, Thompson RP, Anderson RH. Developmental patterning of the myocardium. Anat Rec. 2000;258:319–37.
43. Towbin JA, Lorts A, Jefferies JL. Left ventricular non-compaction cardiomyopathy. Lancet. 2015;386:813–25.
44. Fazio G, Corrado G, Zachara E, Rapezzi C, Sulafa AK, Sutera L, Pizzuto C, Stollberger C, Sormani L, Finsterer J, Benatar A, Di Gesaro G, Cascio C, Cangemi D, Cavusoglu Y, Baumhakel M, Drago F, Carerj S, Pipitone S, Novo S. Ventricular tachycardia in noncompaction of left ventricle: is this a frequent complication? Pacing Clin Electrophysiol. 2007;30:544–6.
45. Sato Y, Matsumoto N, Takahashi H, Imai S, Yoda S, Kasamaki Y, Takayama T, Kunimoto S, Koyama Y, Saito S, Uchiyama T. Cardioverter defibrillator implantation in an adult with isolated noncompaction of the ventricular myocardium. Int J Cardiol. 2006;110:417–9.
46. Guvenc TS, Ilhan E, Alper AT, Eren M. Exercise-induced right ventricular outflow tract tachycardia in a patient with isolated left ventricular noncompaction. ISRN Cardiol. 2011;2011:729040.
47. Derval N, Jais P, O'Neill MD, Haissaguerre M. Apparent idiopathic ventricular tachycardia associated with isolated ventricular noncompaction. Heart Rhythm. 2009;6:385–8.
48. Barra S, Moreno N, Providencia R, Goncalves H, Primo JJ. Incessant slow bundle branch reentrant ventricular tachycardia in a young patient with left ventricular noncompaction. Rev Port Cardiol. 2013;32:523–9.
49. Santoro F, Manuppelli V, Brunetti ND. Multiple morphology ventricular tachycardia in noncompaction cardiomyopathy: multi-modal imaging. Europace. 2013;15:304.
50. Seres L, Lopez J, Larrousse E, Moya A, Pereferrer D, Valle V. Isolated noncompaction left ventricular myocardium and polymorphic ventricular tachycardia. Clin Cardiol. 2003;26:46–8.
51. Junga G, Kneifel S, Von Smekal A, Steinert H, Bauersfeld U. Myocardial ischaemia in children with isolated ventricular non-compaction. Eur Heart J. 1999;20:910–6.
52. Ruberman W, Weinblatt E, Goldberg JD, Frank CW, Shapiro S. Ventricular premature beats and mortality after myocardial infarction. N Engl J Med. 1977;297:750–7.
53. Packer M. Lack of relation between ventricular arrhythmias and sudden death in patients with chronic heart failure. Circulation. 1992;85:I50–6.
54. Van Malderen S, Wijchers S, Akca F, Caliskan K, Szili-Torok T. Mismatch between the origin of premature ventricular complexes and the noncompacted myocardium in patients with noncompaction cardiomyopathy patients: involvement of the conduction system? Ann Noninvasive Electrocardiol. 2017;22:e12394.
55. Engberding R, Bender F. Identification of a rare congenital anomaly of the myocardium by two-dimensional echocardiography: persistence of isolated myocardial sinusoids. Am J Cardiol. 1984;53:1733–4.
56. Steffel J, Duru F. Rhythm disorders in isolated left ventricular noncompaction. Ann Med. 2012;44:101–8.
57. Caliskan K, Balk AH, Jordaens L, Szili-Torok T. Bradycardiomyopathy: the case for a causative relationship between severe sinus bradycardia and heart failure. J Cardiovasc Electrophysiol. 2010;21(7):822–4.
58. Milano A, Vermeer AM, Lodder EM, Barc J, Verkerk AO, Postma AV, van der Bilt IA, Baars MJ, van Haelst PL, Caliskan K, Hoedemaekers YM, Le Scouarnec S, Redon R, Pinto YM, Christiaans I, Wilde AA, Bezzina CR. HCN4 mutations in multiple families with bradycardia and left ventricular noncompaction cardiomyopathy. Coll Cardiol. 2014;64(8):745–56.

59. Paparella G, Capulzini L, de Asmundis C, Francesconi A, Sarkozy A, Chierchia G, Brugada P. Electro-anatomical mapping in a patient with isolated left ventricular non-compaction and left ventricular tachycardia. Europace. 2009;11:1227–9.
60. Sandhu R, Finkelhor RS, Gunawardena DR, Bahler RC. Prevalence and characteristics of left ventricular noncompaction in a community hospital cohort of patients with systolic dysfunction. Echocardiography. 2008;25:8–12.
61. Paterick TE, Gerber TC, Pradhan SR, Lindor NM, Tajik AJ. Left ventricular noncompaction cardiomyopathy: what do we know? Rev Cardiovasc Med. 2010;11:92–9.
62. Jenni R, Wyss CA, Oechslin EN, Kaufmann PA. Isolated ventricular noncompaction is associated with coronary microcirculatory dysfunction. J Am Coll Cardiol. 2002;39:450–4.
63. Desai AS, Fang JC, Maisel WH, Baughman KL. Implantable defibrillators for the prevention of mortality in patients with nonischemic cardiomyopathy: a meta-analysis of randomized controlled trials. JAMA. 2004;292:2874–9.
64. Jenni R, Oechslin E, Schneider J, Attenhofer Jost C, Kaufmann PA. Echocardiographic and pathoanatomical characteristics of isolated left ventricular non-compaction: a step towards classification as a distinct cardiomyopathy. Heart. 2001;86:666–71.
65. Narang R, Cleland JG, Erhardt L, Ball SG, Coats AJ, Cowley AJ, Dargie HJ, Hall AS, Hampton JR, Poole-Wilson PA. Mode of death in chronic heart failure. A request and proposition for more accurate classification. Eur Heart J. 1996;17:1390–403.
66. Murphy RT, Thaman R, Blanes JG, Ward D, Sevdalis E, Papra E, Kiotsekoglou A, Tome MT, Pellerin D, McKenna WJ, Elliott PM. Natural history and familial characteristics of isolated left ventricular non-compaction. Eur Heart J. 2005;26:187–92.
67. Myerburg RJ, Kessler KM, Castellanos A. Sudden cardiac death: epidemiology, transient risk, and intervention assessment. Ann Intern Med. 1993;119:1187–97.

Prevalence and Prevention of Thromboembolic Events in Noncompaction Cardiomyopathy

Attila Nemes

Noncompaction Cardiomyopathy

NCCM is a rare cardiomyopathy with unknown origin which is frequently associated with specific genetic abnormalities [1]. NCCM affects mostly the LV, and hypothesized to be resulting from the arrest of the normal compaction process of the myocardium during foetal development [2]. NCCM is characterized by prominent myocardial trabeculations and deep intertrabecular recesses in the LV cavity [3]. Due to its special phenotype, typical potential complications are heart failure, arrhythmias, and thromboembolic events.

Diagnosis of Noncompaction Cardiomyopathy

The diagnosis of NCCM is mostly based on echocardiography, although its limitations are widely known. For a comprehensive overview, we refer to Chap. 3.

Several echocardiographic criteria are used in the clinical practice, the most known criteria were created by Chin [4], Jenni [5], Stöllberger [6] and Belanger [7]. Although echocardiography is considered to be the gold-standard imaging technology in the diagnosis of NCCM, Diwadkar et al. found that echocardiography fails to detect NCCM morphology/hypertrabeculation in a significant number of a cohort of patients on cardiac magnetic resonance imaging (cMRI) in a recent study [8]. These findings suggest ambiguous results in the diagnosis of NCCM, making the real prevalence of NCCM more complicated.

A. Nemes (✉)
2nd Department of Medicine and Cardiology Center, Faculty of Medicine, Albert Szent-Györgyi Clinical Center, University of Szeged, Szeged, Hungary
e-mail: nemes.attila@med.u-szeged.hu

© Springer Nature Switzerland AG 2019
K. Caliskan et al. (eds.), *Noncompaction Cardiomyopathy*,
https://doi.org/10.1007/978-3-030-17720-1_6

Case 1: A Patient with Noncompaction Cardiomyopathy

A case of a 50-year-old female patient is presented. Muscular ventricular septal defect and persistent foramen ovale are present in her medical history with chronic heart failure originating from familiar NCCM. At the age of 40, the patient suffered a cerebrovascular accident with mild hemiparesis. Oral anticoagulation was prescribed along with optimization of her heart failure medication. Four years later, there was a suspected transient ischaemic attack. In 2015, a VDD-ICD was implanted for primary prevention for cardiac death; the intervention was complicated with right ventricular perforation, pericardial effusion and dislocation of the VDD lead. Recently, her functional class was in New York Heart Association functional grade I, routine two-dimensional Doppler echocardiography confirmed reduced LV systolic function with ejection fraction of approximately 30–35% and grade 2 diastolic dysfunction (E/E′ proved to be 14.3) without significant valvular regurgitation or stenosis (Figs. 6.1 and 6.2). Wall motion analysis confirmed diffuse LV hypokinesis with inferior basal and midventricular akinesis (wall motion score index = 2.24), The right ventricular function proved to be normal. Electrocardiography (ECG) did not confirm significant arrhythmia (Fig. 6.3).

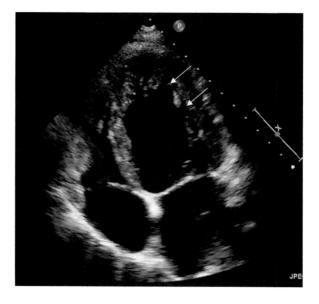

Fig. 6.1 Routine 2-dimensional echocardiography demonstrating hypertrabecularization of the LV apex with intertrabecular recesses (see white arrows)

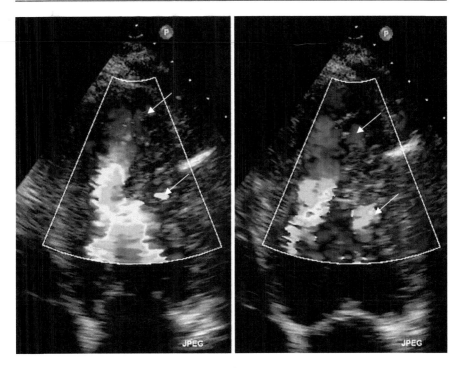

Fig. 6.2 Colour Doppler echocardiographic images demonstrating intertrabecular recesses (see white arrows)

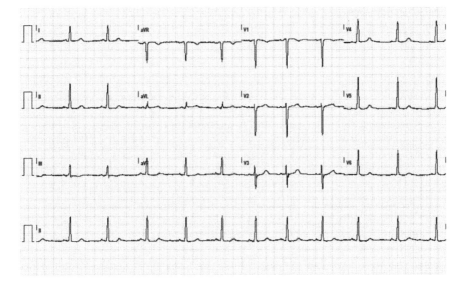

Fig. 6.3 Routine electrocardiography demonstrating normofrequent sinus rhythm without significant arrhythmia or conductance disorder

Prevalence of Noncompaction Cardiomyopathy

The true prevalence of NCCM in the general population would be determined based on population-based echocardiographic screening. However, there are no population-based studies to determine the real prevalence of NCCM [1]. The first prospective and large echocardiography-based study to determine the real prevalence of NCCM has just been published [1]. This prospective case-control study included all subjects who underwent a transthoracic echocardiogram in an academic center within one-year [1]. From 10,857 echocardiograms performed, 26 cases of NCCM were detected giving an estimated prevalence of 0.24% for this cohort [1]. Most patients (77%) had ≤50% LV ejection fraction in higher ages. When cases with dilated cardiomyopathies of different aetiologies were analysed, 6.8% of the cases showed NCCM with EF <50%. When only those patients with idiopathic dilated cardiomyopathy were included, the estimated prevalence of NCCM was 24%. When LV noncompaction was detected only incidentally in an otherwise healthy and asymptomatic population with normal ejection fraction, the prevalence was 0.05% [1]. In a recent study by Ivanov et al., a cohort of 700 patients referred for cMRI underwent diagnostic assessment for NCCM by four separate imaging criteria referenced by their authors as Petersen, Stacey, Jacquier, and Captur, with a NCCM prevalence of 39%, 23%, 25% and 3%, respectively [9]. In the childhood, large paediatric studies have found NCCM to be the most common form of unclassified cardiomyopathies [10, 11].

Prevalence of Thromboembolic Events in Noncompaction Cardiomyopathy

There are conflicting results about the prevalence of the most feared NCCM-related complications, the thromboembolic events in NCCM, but these complications seem to be not uncommon in NCCM. Cardiac emboli are theorized to result from thrombus formation within the intertrabecular recesses, but reduced systolic function predispose to thrombosis as well. The higher risk of arrhythmias, including atrial fibrillation (AF) is also considerable source of the evolution of thromboembolism in NCCM [12]. The other important risk factors for thromboembolic events are previous thromboembolic events, hypertension, coagulopathy, etc. [13, 14]. According to the literature, stroke and embolism occur in at least 15% of patients with NCCM due to above mentioned reasons [14]. However, it should also be considered that in cases of NCCM with AF, thrombi may not only be derived from the intertrabecular spaces but also from the left atrium or left atrial appendage [15]. The overall thromboembolic annualized event rate is not different as compared to heart failure patients or subjects with other cardiomyopathies [16].

Anticoagulant Treatment for Stroke Prevention

Anticoagulant Treatment for Stroke Prevention in General Cardiac Patients

Oral anticoagulant therapy (OAC) prevents the majority of ischaemic strokes in patient with AF and is confirmed to prolong life [17]. Men with a CHA_2DS_2-VASc of 2 or more and women with a CHA_2DS_2-VASc score of 3 or more are suggested to benefit from OAC. Therefore, OAC should be considered from a CHA_2DS_2-VASc of 1 in men and 2 in women considering the potential adverse events, including bleeding risks and the patients' preference. Vitamin K antagonists (VKA), the first anticoagulants used in patients with AF were confirmed to reduce the risk of stroke by two-thirds and to reduce mortality by 25% compared with control. VKA therapy is limited by the narrow therapeutic range of VKAs, the need for close monitoring and potential dose adjustments. Non-vitamin K type oral anticoagulants (NOACs), including the direct thrombin inhibitor dabigatran and the factor Xa inhibitors, apixaban, edoxaban and rivaroxaban, are suitable alternative treatment options to VKAs for stroke prevention in patients with AF. NOACs have a predictable effect (onset and offset), no regular laboratory test is required to test the efficacy of NOACs. NOACs are recommended in preference to VKAs or acetylsalicylic acid in AF patients with a previous stroke [17].

In patients with heart failure with reduced ejection fraction (HFrEF) or preserved EF (HFpEF) however, there is no evidence that the use of warfarin reduces mortality and morbidity as compared to placebo or acetylsalicylic acid [18]. Therefore, new studies with NOACs in patients with HFrEF are ongoing.

Anticoagulation Therapy for Stroke Prevention in Noncompaction Cardiomyopathy Patients

It is generally recommended to those presenting with antecedent of systemic embolism, presence of cardiac thrombus and AF and ventricular systolic dysfunction [19]. Unfortunately, due to its rarity, evidence-based recommendations for preventing thromboembolic events in isolated NCCM have not been established. It is still not clear under which conditions NCCM patients should be clearly anticoagulated for primary prophylaxis of stroke or embolism. According to the latest literature on how to use anticoagulants in LV noncompaction, the recommendations are the following:

- If NCCM is associated with AF, the usefulness of anticoagulants seem to be reasonable by reducing thromboembolic rate including vitamin K-antagonists (VKA) and new oral anticoagulants (NOAC) [15, 20].
- If NCCM is associated with a history of previous stroke and embolism, VKA or NOAC should be considered [15, 20].

- If NCCM is associated with systolic dysfunction and sinus rhythm, no significant overall difference could be demonstrated in the primary outcome between treatment with VKA and high dose acetylsalicylic acid [21]. Anticoagulant treatment in these patients without history of previous thromboembolism is still on debate. Given the deep intertrabecular recesses and probably slurred local slow flows, historically the NCCM patients has been always considered as high-risk patients for thromboembolic events. Therefore, till we have more clear and specific evidence, we advise in general anticoagulation therapy in NCCM patients with significant LV dysfunction (i.e. empirically LVEF <40%) and/or heart failure.

To understand the potential indications of anticoagulation therapy in noncompaction cardiomyopathy, here some cases are presented.

Case 2: A Patient with Noncompaction Cardiomyopathy with Atrial Fibrillation

A case of a 35-year-old male patient is presented. His medical history started with palpitations at the age of 32, when electrocardiography (ECG) showed sinus rhythm. Routine transthoracic Doppler echocardiography revealed mildly enlarged LV and atria without significant valvular alterations. LV ejection fraction was 60%, grade 2 diastolic dysfunction could be confirmed with normal RV sizes and function. With Doppler echocardiography, deeply perfused intertrabecular recesses could be demonstrated suggesting NCCM (Fig. 6.4). The patients did not show any signs of heart failure. But Holter ECG showed paroxysmal atrial fibrillation (Fig. 6.5). Therefore, oral anticoagulation was initiated.

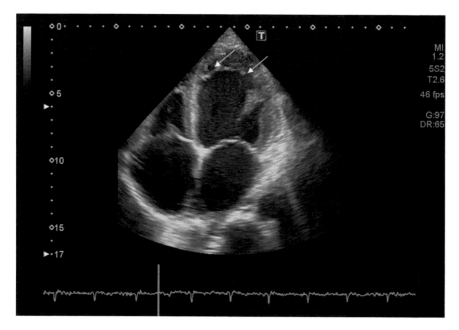

Fig. 6.4 Routine 2-dimensional echocardiography of a 35-year-old male demonstrating hypertrabecularization of the LV apex with intertrabecular recesses (see white arrows)

Fig. 6.5 Routine electrocardiography demonstrating high frequency atrial fibrillation

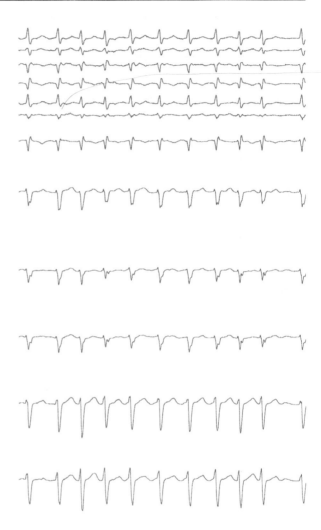

Case 3: A Patient with Noncompaction Cardiomyopathy with Systolic Dysfunction

A 58-year-old male presented with shortness of breath on exertion and atypical chest pain. His past medical history consisted of mild mitral regurgitation, hyperlipidemia, and osteoporosis. His present symptoms started 1 month ago, with chest X-ray showing cardiomegaly. ECG showed sinus rhythm with normal heart rate (Fig. 6.6). Two-dimensional transthoracic echocardiography revealed signs of LV hypertrophy with diffuse myocardial lesion and reduced LV function (ejection fraction: 37%) could be demonstrated by. But, detailed echocardiographic evaluation of the thickened myocardial walls showed hypertrabecularization of the LV apex and

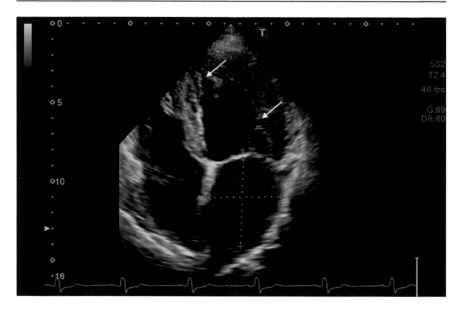

Fig. 6.6 Routine 2-dimensional echocardiography demonstrating hypertrabecularization of the LV apex with intertrabecular recesses

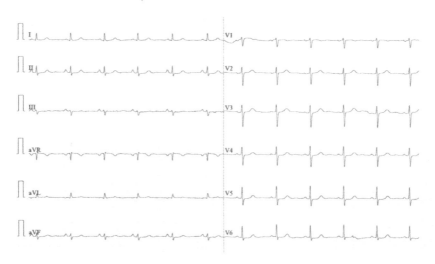

Fig. 6.7 Routine electrocardiography demonstrating normofrequent sinus rhythm without significant arrhythmia or conductance disorder

septum rather than LV hypertrophy. Colour Doppler echocardiography confirmed intertrabecular recesses, confirming the diagnosis of NCCM (Fig. 6.7). Given the significant LV dysfunction with a LVEF <40%, we prescribed empirically oral anti-coagulation along with ACE-inibitor and beta-blocker.

Conclusions

Thromboembolic events are relatively common in NCCM patients. Unfortunately, due to its rarity and relatively young disease entity, evidence-based recommendations for preventing thromboembolic events in NCCM have not been established. In patients with atrial fibrillation or flutter oral anticoagulation including vitamin K antagonists (VKA) and new oral anticoagulants (NOAC), seem to be reasonable to reduce thromboembolic rate. In case of a history of previous stroke and thromboembolism, VKA or NOAC use is according the current clinical insights beyond any doubt. In NCCM patient with an systolic dysfunction, but sinus rhythm, overall benefit of preventive oral anticoagulation is yet to be demonstrated. Further research for evidence-based guidelines are highly needed.

References

1. Ronderos R, Avegliano G, Borelli E, Kuschnir P, Castro F, Sanchez G, Perea G, Corneli M, Zanier MM, Andres S, Aranda A, Conde D, Trivi M. Estimation of prevalence of the left ventricular noncompaction among adults. Am J Cardiol. 2016;118:901–5.
2. Udeoji DU, Philip KJ, Morrissey RP, Phan A, Schwarz ER. Left ventricular noncompaction cardiomyopathy: updated review. Ther Adv Cardiovasc Dis. 2013;7:260–73.
3. Ikeda U, Minamisawa M, Koyama J. Isolated left ventricular non-compaction cardiomyopathy in adults. J Cardiol. 2015;65:91–7.
4. Chin TK, Perloff JK, Williams RG, Jue K, Mohrmann R. Isolated noncompaction of left ventricular myocardium. A study of eight cases. Circulation. 1990;82:507–13.
5. Jenni R, Oechslin E, Schneider J, Attenhofer Jost C, Kaufmann PA. Echocardiographic and pathoanatomical characteristics of isolated left ventricular non-compaction: a step towards classification as a distinct cardiomyopathy. Heart. 2001;86(6):666–71.
6. Stöllberger C, Finsterer J. Left ventricular hypertrabeculation/noncompaction. J Am Soc Echocardiogr. 2004;17:91–100.
7. Belanger AR, Miller MA, Donthireddi UR, Najovits AJ, Goldman ME. New classification scheme of left ventricular noncompaction and correlation with ventricular performance. Am J Cardiol. 2008;102:92–6.
8. Diwadkar S, Nallamshetty L, Rojas C, Athienitis A, Declue C, Cox C, Patel A, Chae SH. Echocardiography fails to detect left ventricular noncompaction in a cohort of patients with noncompaction on cardiac magnetic resonance imaging. Clin Cardiol. 2017;40:364–9.
9. Ivanov A, Dabiesingh DS, Bhumireddy GP, Mohamed A, Asfour A, Briggs WM, Ho J, Khan SA, Grossman A, Klem I, Sacchi TJ, Heitner JF. Prevalence and prognostic significance of left ventricular noncompaction in patients referred for cardiac magnetic resonance imaging. Circ Cardiovasc Imaging. 2017;10:e006174.
10. Nugent AW, Daubeney PE, Chondros P, Carlin JB, Cheung M, Wilkinson LC, Davis AM, Kahler SG, Chow CW, Wilkinson JL, Weintraub RG, National Australian Childhood Cardiomyopathy Study. The epidemiology of childhood cardiomyopathy in Australia. N Engl J Med. 2003;348:1639–46.
11. Pignatelli RH, McMahon CJ, Dreyer WJ, Denfield SW, Price J, Belmont JW, Craigen WJ, Wu J, El Said H, Bezold LI, Clunie S, Fembach S, Bowles NE, Towbin JA. Clinical characterization of left ventricular noncompaction in children: a relatively common form of cardiomyopathy. Circulation. 2003;108:2672–8.
12. Miyake CY, Kim JJ. Arrhythmias in left ventricular noncompaction. Card Electrophysiol Clin. 2015;7:319–30.

13. Thavendiranathan P, Dahiya A, Phelan D, Desai MY, Tang WH. Isolated left ventricular non-compaction controversies in diagnostic criteria, adverse outcomes and management. Heart. 2013;99:681–9.
14. Stöllberger C, Blazek G, Dobias C, Hanafin A, Wegner C, Finsterer J. Frequency of stroke and embolism in left ventricular hypertrabeculation/noncompaction. Am J Cardiol. 2011;108:1021–3.
15. Finsterer J, Stöllberger C. Primary prophylactic anticoagulation is mandatory if noncompaction is associated with atrial fibrillation or heart failure. Int J Cardiol. 2015;184:268–9.
16. Rooms I, Dujardin K, De Sutter J. Non-compaction cardiomyopathy: a genetically and clinically heterogeneous disorder. Acta Cardiol. 2015;70:625–31.
17. Kirchhof P, Benussi S, Kotecha D, Ahlsson A, Atar D, Casadei B, Castella M, Diener HC, Heidbuchel H, Hendriks J, Hindricks G, Manolis AS, Oldgren J, Popescu BA, Schotten U, Van Putte B, Vardas P, Agewall S, Camm J, Baron Esquivias G, Budts W, Carerj S, Casselman F, Coca A, De Caterina R, Deftereos S, Dobrev D, Ferro JM, Filippatos G, Fitzsimons D, Gorenek B, Guenoun M, Hohnloser SH, Kolh P, Lip GY, Manolis A, McMurray J, Ponikowski P, Rosenhek R, Ruschitzka F, Savelieva I, Sharma S, Suwalski P, Tamargo JL, Taylor CJ, Van Gelder IC, Voors AA, Windecker S, Zamorano JL, Zeppenfeld K. 2016 ESC Guidelines for the management of atrial fibrillation developed in collaboration with EACTS. Eur Heart J. 2016;37:2893–962.
18. Ponikowski P, Voors AA, Anker SD, Bueno H, Cleland JG, Coats AJ, Falk V, González-Juanatey JR, Harjola VP, Jankowska EA, Jessup M, Linde C, Nihoyannopoulos P, Parissis JT, Pieske B, Riley JP, Rosano GM, Ruilope LM, Ruschitzka F, Rutten FH, van der Meer P, Members A/TF, Reviewers D. 2016 ESC Guidelines for the diagnosis and treatment of acute and chronic heart failure: The Task Force for the diagnosis and treatment of acute and chronic heart failure of the European Society of Cardiology (ESC). Developed with the special contribution of the Heart Failure Association (HFA) of the ESC. Eur J Heart Fail. 2016;18:891–975.
19. Tavares de Melo MD, de Araújo Filho JA, Parga Filho JR, de Lima CR, Mady C, Kalil-Filho R, Salemi VM. Noncompaction cardiomyopathy: a substrate for a thromboembolic event. BMC Cardiovasc Disord. 2015;15:7.
20. Erath JW, Hohnloser SH. Anticoagulation in atrial fibrillation: current evidence and guideline recommendations. Herz. 2018;43(1):2–10.
21. Homma S, Thompson JL, Pullicino PM, Levin B, Freudenberger RS, Teerlink JR, Ammon SE, Graham S, Sacco RL, Mann DL, Mohr JP, Massie BM, Labovitz AJ, Anker SD, Lok DJ, Ponikowski P, Estol CJ, Lip GY, Di Tullio MR, Sanford AR, Mejia V, Gabriel AP, del Valle ML, Buchsbaum R; WARCEF Investigators. Warfarin and aspirin in patients with heart failure and sinus rhythm. N Engl J Med. 2012;366:1859–69.

Noncompaction Cardiomyopathy in Childhood

7

Jeffrey A. Towbin, Kaitlin Ryan, and Jason Goldberg

Noncompaction cardiomyopathy (NCCM), also called left ventricular noncompaction (LVNC), a classified form of cardiomyopathy, is a genetic disease characterized by excessive and unusual trabeculations within the mature left ventricle (LV). NCCM has been considered to be a developmental failure of the heart to form fully the compact myocardium during the later stages of cardiac development. Clinically and pathologically, NCCM is characterized by a spongy morphological appearance of the myocardium occurring primarily in the LV with the abnormal trabeculations typically being most evident in the apical and midlateral-inferior portions of the LV. The right ventricle (RV) may also be affected alone or in conjunction with the LV. In NCCM, in addition to the regional presence of prominent trabeculae and inter-trabecular recesses in the LV, thickening of the myocardium in 2 distinct layers composed of compacted and non-compacted myocardium is also classically noted. It may be associated with left ventricular dilation or hypertrophy, systolic and/or diastolic dysfunction, atrial enlargement, or various forms of congenital heart disease. The myocardium in NCCM may demonstrate normal or abnormal systolic or diastolic function and the size, thickness or function may change unexpectedly ("undulating phenotype"). Affected individuals are at risk of left or right ventricular failure, or both. Heart failure symptoms can be exercise-induced or persistent at rest, but many patients are asymptomatic. Chronically treated patients sometimes present acutely with decompensated heart failure. Other life-threatening risks are ventricular arrhythmias and atrioventricular block, presenting clinically as syncope,

J. A. Towbin (✉) · K. Ryan · J. Goldberg
The Heart Institute, Le Bonheur Children's Hospital,
Memphis, TN, USA

Cardiomyopathy Program, St. Jude Children's Research Hospital,
Memphis, TN, USA

Division of Pediatric Cardiology, University of Tennessee Health Science Center, Memphis,
TN, USA
e-mail: jtowbin1@uthsc.edu

© Springer Nature Switzerland AG 2019
K. Caliskan et al. (eds.), *Noncompaction Cardiomyopathy*,
https://doi.org/10.1007/978-3-030-17720-1_7

and sudden death. Genetic inheritance arises in at least 30–50% of patients, NCCM is thought to occur in approximately 1 per 7000 live births. It occurs in newborns, young children and adults, with the worst reported outcomes seen in infants, particularly those with associated systemic disease and metabolic derangement. In some families, a consistent phenotype of NCCM is seen in affected relatives but quite commonly individuals with features of NCCM are found in families where other affected relatives have typical hypertrophic cardiomyopathy, dilated cardiomyopathy, or restrictive cardiomyopathy. Mutations in ~15 genes have been implicated and include cytoskeletal, sarcomeric, and ion channel genes, with sarcomere-encoding genes being most common. In the case of NCCM with congenital heart disease, disturbance of the Notch or Wnt signaling pathways appear to be part of a "final common pathway" for this form of the disease. In addition, disrupted mitochondrial function and metabolic abnormalities have a causal role as well. Treatments focus on improvement of cardiac efficiency and reduction of mechanical stress in those with systolic dysfunction. Further, arrhythmia therapy and implantation of an automatic implantable cardioverter-defibrillator (ICD) for prevention of sudden death are mainstays of treatment when deemed necessary and appropriate. Patients with NCCM associated with congenital heart disease commonly require surgical or catheter-based interventions. Despite progress in diagnosis and treatment over the past 10–15 years, understanding of the disorder and outcomes continue to need further improvement.

Introduction

Noncompaction cardiomyopathy (NCCM), also called left ventricular noncompaction cardiomyopathy (NCCM), first described by Grant [1] in 1926, is a heterogeneous myocardial disorder characterized by prominent trabeculae, intra-trabecular recesses, and left ventricular myocardium having two distinct layers: compacted and noncompacted myocardium [2–4]. Continuity exists between the left ventricular cavity and deep intra-trabecular recesses, both of which are filled with blood, and there is no evidence of communication to the epicardial coronary artery system [5, 6]. Although NCCM primarily affects the left ventricle, isolated right ventricular and biventricular noncompaction also occurs [7–9]. Imaging and pathology evaluation demonstrates NCCM to be characterized by a spongy morphological appearance of the left ventricular myocardium with abnormal trabeculations typically most evident in the left ventricular apex as we and others have previously reported [3, 10]. The LV free wall may also be affected but the interventricular septum is rarely affected, with the exception of the apical portion of the interventricular septum. The American Heart Association "Scientific Statement on Classification of Cardiomyopathies" formally classified NCCM as a distinct cardiomyopathy in 2006 [11].

NCCM has been called by a variety of names including spongy myocardium, fetal myocardium, noncompaction of the left ventricular myocardium, hypertrabeculation syndrome, and left ventricular noncompaction, among others [2, 3, 6, 10–16]. The genesis of NCCM has been speculated to represent arrest of the final stage of myocardial morphogenesis (myocardial compaction) [5, 6, 17–22]. However, this does not explain the fact that multiple forms of NCCM occur and these include primary myocardial forms of NCCM, a form associated with arrhythmias, and NCCM associated with congenital heart disease, including septal defects, right heart obstructive abnormalities including pulmonic stenosis and Ebstein's anomaly, hypoplastic left heart syndrome, and others [10, 12, 23–29]. In all forms of NCCM, we and others have shown that metabolic derangements may be notable, particularly in newborns and infants [10, 30, 31].

Pathology of Noncompaction Cardiomyopathy

In the early embryo, the heart is a loose interwoven mesh of muscle fibers [5, 6, 17, 19–21]. The developing myocardium gradually condenses, and the large spaces within the trabecular meshwork disappear, condensing and compacting the ventricular myocardium and solidifying the endocardial surfaces. Trabecular compaction is normally more complete in the left ventricular than in the right ventricular myocardium, and therefore right ventricular trabeculations (albeit small) are normally seen in the mature heart. Hence, this compacting pathway failure is thought to occur due to arrest of endomyocardial morphogenesis, causing postnatal NCCM [5, 6, 17, 19–21]. The gross pathologic appearance of NCCM is characterized by numerous excessively prominent trabeculations with deep intra-trabecular recesses resembling the right ventricular endomyocardial morphology. Histologically, the recesses and their troughs are lined with endothelium. Zones of fibrous and elastic tissue may be scattered on the endocardial surfaces with extension into the recesses. The coronary arterial circulation is usually normal; extramural myocardial blood supply is not believed to play a role in these abnormalities [32]. Intramural perfusion, however, could be adversely affected by the prominent trabeculations and intra-trabecular recesses, particularly in the subendocardium, causing subendocardial ischemia. Although there is no clear evidence that subendocardial ischemia is causative of NCCM, it is possible that an ischemic insult to critical signaling pathways between the myocardium and the endocardium could impact ventricular trabeculation formation and resorption [33, 34]. During cardiogenesis, the cardiac jelly plays an important role in the interaction between these two layers. Whether ischemia could result in a disruption or modification of signaling pathways is not clear [35]. In addition, there is no definitive evidence of subendocardial fibrosis using cardiac MRI and late gadolinium enhancement. The endomyocardial morphology of NCCM also lends itself to development of mural thrombi within ischemia playing a significant role in the clinical course of patients with NCCM, although in some patients the recesses which can embolize, causing a stroke or coronary obstruction [3, 10, 14, 36, 37]. Arrhythmias may also occur and consists of either tachy- or bradyarrhythmias, and these arrhythmias impact outcome [24, 25, 38, 39].

Incidence of Noncompaction Cardiomyopathy

Although NCCM has been considered rare by some authors, and the incidence and prevalence of NCCM is uncertain, it appears to be the third most commonly diagnosed cardiomyopathy. NCCM is thought to occur in approximately 1 per 7000 live births. It occurs in newborns, young children and adults, with the worst reported outcomes seen in infants, particularly those with associated systemic disease and metabolic derangement. Ritter et al. [40] reported the prevalence of isolated NCCM to be 0.05% of all adult echocardiographic examinations in a large institution while Aras et al. [41] reported the prevalence to be <0.14% of adults referred for echocardiograms. In contrast, Sandhu et al. demonstrated a 3.7% prevalence of definite or probable NCCM by echocardiography in adults with left ventricular ejection fractions (EF) ≤45% and 0.26% prevalence for all patients referred for echocardiography [42]. Among heart failure patients, the prevalence of NCCM has been reported as 3–4% [43, 44]. Most recently, Ronderos et al. reported a on a total of 10,857 adult patients who underwent echocardiography [45]. They showed that 2931 (27%) were normal, while NCCM was found in 26 patients (prevalence = 0.24%). In this cohort, 16 patients were women, mean age of 52.6 years. Patients were divided into 2 groups; group A: ejection fraction (EF) <50% (n = 20) and group B: normal systolic function (n = 6). Among abnormal studies, 294 (2.7%) were associated with a dilated cardiomyopathy (DCM). In patients with NCCM, and EF <50% comprised 6.8% of DCM (20 of 294) and 24% (20 of 75) of patients with idiopathic DC (p < 0.0001). Group A patients were older and they have less presence of women (both p < 0.05). In conclusion, the prevalence of NCCM in a population assessed for cardiovascular diseases is low. In contrast, it is very high in the subgroup of patients with idiopathic DCM. The group of patients with NCCM and normal LVEF is younger and with a higher presence of women than those with NCCM and depressed LVEF. Coincidence between operators is very good for the identification of echocardiographic criteria (Tables 7.1 and 7.2).

These wide variations in the reported incidence and prevalence are likely dependent on clinical recognition of the disease and the diagnosis of NCCM is now becoming more frequent. This is most likely due to an increased awareness of the disease, and the improved imaging technology, as well as recommendations for screening at-risk family members who also have the NCCM phenotype due to its hereditary nature.

Table 7.1 Genetic causes of left ventricular noncompaction

Gene	Gene name	Protein type
ACTC1	α-Cardiac Actin	Sarcomere thin filament
CASQ2	Cardiac Calsequestrin 2	Calcium homeostasis
DTNA	α-Dystrobrevin	Cytoskeletal protein
DYS	Dystrophin	Cytoskeletal protein
GLA	α-Galactosidase	Glycoside hydrolase
LDB3	LIM-domain binding 3	Z-disk protein
LMNA	Lamin A/C	Nuclear membrane protein
MIB1	Mindbomb homolog 1	E3 ubiquitin ligase
MYBPC3	Myosin Binding Protein C	Sarcomere thick filament
MYH7	β-Myosin Heavy Chain 7	Sarcomere thick filament
Nkx2-5	Nkx2-5	Transcription factor
TAZ	Tafazzin	Phospholipid transacylase
TNNT2	Cardiac Troponin T, type 2	Sarcomere thin filament

Table 7.2 Mouse models of left ventricular noncompaction

Mutant gene	Mutant type	Clinical features
Fkbp1a	Fkbp1a-deficient	NCCM, VSD
Bmp10	Bmp10-overexpression	NCCM, VSD
Smad7	Smad7-deficient	NCCM, HF, VSD, RVOTO, Arrhythmia
NF-ATc	NF-ATc-deficient	NCCM, HF, VSD, RVOTO
Jarid2/Jumonji	Jarid2-deficient	NCCM, VSD, DORV
TAZ	TAZ-knockdown	NCCM
MIB1	MIB1-deficient	NCCM, RVNC, DCM, HF
Nkx2-5	Nkx2-5-deficient	NCCM, DCM, HF, AVB

Clinical Features and Diagnosis of Noncompaction Cardiomyopathy

The clinical presentation of NCCM is highly variable. It occurs at any age, can range from asymptomatic to end-stage heart failure, or be associated with lethal arrhythmias, sudden cardiac death and/or thrombo-embolic events [2–4, 7–10, 12–14, 46, 47]. A high percentage of patients are asymptomatic, being identified seren-dipitously by echocardiogram after referral due to a murmur or for familial screening. Some patients with NCCM present with clinically significant arrhythmias or conduction system disease as discussed below. Reports regarding outcome in children and adults have been inconsistent, with some demonstrating poor outcomes and others having a low percent of death or transplantation. For instance, Ichida et al. [14] found good survival and limited symptoms in their childhood patients while Chin et al. [2] reported three deaths in the eight children studied. Our group demonstrated poor outcome in neonates but excellent outcomes in older children, with a 75% five-year survival free of death or transplantation. The neonates that died all had systemic disease (mitochondrial or other metabolic disorders).

Adult clinical studies have consistently described a high risk of ventricular tachyarrhythmias and sudden cardiac death in NCCM, with up to 47% of adults (and 75% of symptomatic patients) dying within six years of presentation [4, 24, 37–39]. More recent reports on an adult cohort, however, have shown a more benign natural history, with lower risk for (malignant) ventricular arrhythmias [48]. Bhatia et al. reviewed published studies of 241 adults with isolated NCCM diagnosed by echocardiographic criteria followed for a mean duration of 39 months [49] and reported an annualized event rate of 4% for cardiovascular deaths, 6.2% for cardiovascular death and its surrogates (transplantation, appropriate implantable cardioverter-defibrillator shocks), and 8.6% for all cardiovascular events (death, stroke, implantable cardioverter-defibrillator shocks, transplantation). Familial NCCM was identified in 30% of first-degree relatives of index cases screened by echocardiography [49]. Brescia et al. retrospectively reviewed all children diagnosed with left ventricular noncompaction at a Children's Hospital from January 1990 to January 2009. Patients with congenital cardiac lesions were excluded [50]. Two hundred forty-two children were diagnosed with isolated left ventricular noncompaction over the study period.

Thirty-one (12.8%) died, and 13 (5.4%) received a transplant. One hundred fifty (62%) presented with or developed cardiac dysfunction. The presence of cardiac dysfunction was strongly associated with mortality (hazard ratio, 11; P < 0.001). ECG abnormalities were present in 87%, with ventricular hypertrophy and repolarization abnormalities occurring most commonly. Repolarization abnormalities were associated with increased mortality (hazard ratio, 2.1; P = 0.02). Eighty children (33.1%) had an arrhythmia, and those with arrhythmias had increased mortality (hazard ratio, 2.8; P = 0.002). Forty-two (17.4%) had ventricular tachycardia, with 5 presenting with resuscitated sudden cardiac death. In total, there were 15 cases of sudden cardiac death in the cohort (6.2%). Nearly all patients with sudden death (14 of 15) had abnormal cardiac dimensions or cardiac dysfunction. No patient with normal cardiac dimensions and function without preceding arrhythmias died. Preceding cardiac dysfunction or ventricular arrhythmias was associated with increased mortality. The precise substrate for malignant ventricular arrhythmias in NCCM patients remains unknown, however [50].

Subtypes of Noncompaction Cardiomyopathy

Although the diagnosis of NCCM has focused primarily on the identification and description of trabeculations, other features are critical to defining the specific type of NCCM. Most reports of NCCM focus on "isolated NCCM" or NCCM with congenital heart disease. However, both the "isolated" and congenital heart disease-associated forms have a wide spectrum of features [10, 51, 52]. This "lumping" instead of "splitting" approach has several disadvantages, particularly when considering outcomes and therapies. At least eight different NCCM phenotypes appear to exist, all having different outcomes (Figs. 7.1a–f and 7.2a–b). A brief description of the subtypes that we have developed [10] is described below:

1. *"Benign" Form of NCCM or "LVNC"*: This subtype is characterized by normal left ventricular size and wall thickness with preserved systolic and diastolic function. This subtype accounts for up to ~35% of NCCM patients and is a predictor of good outcome in the absence of significant arrhythmias [52]. It is this patient population that has led to statements by mostly adult cardiologists that NCCM does not represent a cardiomyopathy and is a benign and normal variant. One possibility for this conclusion is that the more severe forms of NCCM tend to occur in childhood and these patients are either successfully treated, transplanted or die and, therefore, do not present to adult cardiologists with symptomatic disease. This subtype appears to have the same outcome as the normal population.

2. *NCCM with Arrhythmias*: This subtype is defined by preserved systolic function with normal left ventricular size and wall thickness but has evidence of underlying arrhythmias, usually identified at the time of diagnosis. We and others have shown that the presence of ventricular arrhythmias is an independent risk factor of mortality, many going unrecognized by current surveillance techniques [10, 24, 25, 37, 38, 52–56]. This subtype appears to have a worse outcome compared to the normal population or those with similar forms of rhythm disturbance.

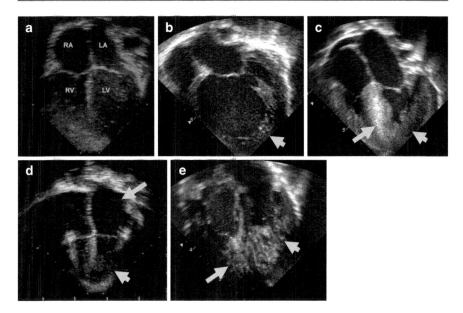

Fig. 7.1 Phenotypes of NCCM on two dimensional echocardiographic four-chamber views. (**a**) Benign form of NCCM in a 12 year old; Note, trabeculations and intra-trabecular recesses seen at the apex of the left ventricle; (**b**) Dilated cardiomyopathy form of NCCM in a 6 year old. Note the dilated LV and hyper-trabeculation of the apex and free wall (arrow); (**c**) Hypertrophic cardiomyopathy form of NCCM in a 14 month old. Note the asymmetric septal hypertrophy (arrow, left), dilated atria caused by severe diastolic dysfunction, and apical hyper-trabeculation (arrow, right); (**d**) Restrictive cardiomyopathy form of NCCM in a 5 year old. Note the dilated atria (top arrow) in the absence of atrioventricular valve regurgitation, and the apical hyper-trabeculation (bottom arrow); LV hypertrophy is absent in this heart; (**e**) Biventricular cardiomyopathy form of NCCM in a 16 year old. Note the heavy trabeculations in both the LV and RV; Arrows, trabeculations in both ventricles

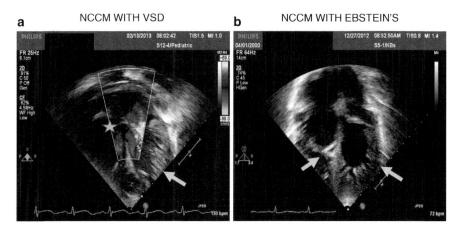

Fig. 7.2 NCCM associated with congenital heart disease. (**a**) NCCM in association with congenital heart disease in a 3 year old with a ventricular septal defect (VSD); star, ventricular septal defect with color Doppler; and LV hyper-trabeculation (arrow); (**b**) NCCM in association with Ebstein's anomaly in a newborn infant. Note the displacement of the tricuspid valve, consistent with Ebstein's anomaly; Arrow left, tricuspid valve displacement with ventricular atrialization. Note LV hyper-trabeculation (arrow, right)

3. *Dilated Cardiomyopathy Form of NCCM*: This subtype is characterized by concomitant left ventricular dilation and systolic dysfunction [3, 10, 14, 42, 43, 48,
52]. During the clinical course of this subtype, an "undulating phenotype" may
present in which the left ventricle may become smaller with some wall hypertrophy and improved function before reverting to the dilated subtype [3]. This
subtype appears to have a similar outcome compared to those with a similar
degree of dilated cardiomyopathy, except in neonates and infants, who have a
worse outcome.

4. *Hypertrophic Cardiomyopathy Form of NCCM*: This subtype is characterized by
left ventricular thickening, usually with asymmetric septal hypertrophy, in addition to diastolic dysfunction and hypercontractile systolic function [10, 52]. In
some cases left ventricular dilation with systolic dysfunction can occur late in
the course of the disease. This subtype appears to have a similar outcome compared to the normal population or those with similar degree of hypertrophic
cardiomyopathy.

5. *Hypertrophic and Dilated Cardiomyopathy Form of NCCM*: This subtype, also
known as a *mixed phenotype*, is characterized by left ventricular thickening, dilation, and depressed systolic function at presentation. This phenotype has
increased risk of mortality and, in pediatric patients, is commonly associated
with metabolic or mitochondrial disease [3, 10, 30, 52]. This form is the most
common of the "undulating" types and most typically ends as a dilated left ventricle with poor function and heart failure [3, 10]. This subtype does worse than
patients with mixed phenotypes for other causes, such as "burned out" forms of
hypertrophic cardiomyopathy.

6. *Restrictive Cardiomyopathy Form of NCCM*: This rare form of NCCM is characterized by left atrial or biatrial dilation and diastolic dysfunction. This phenotype mimics the clinical behavior of restrictive cardiomyopathy with a similarly
poor outcome, typically due to arrhythmia-related sudden cardiac events or, less
commonly, heart failure with preserved ejection fraction [10, 52]. This subtype
appears to have a similar outcome compared to those with similar forms of
restrictive cardiomyopathy.

7. *Right ventricular or Biventricular Cardiomyopathy Form of NCCM*: This subtype is characterized by hyper-trabeculation of both the right ventricle and left
ventricle. There are no recognized diagnostic criteria for right ventricular noncompaction (RVNC). Previous reports have suggested applying left ventricular
diagnostic criteria to the right ventricle [57]. We have relied on a finding of very
heavy right ventricular trabeculations and a severe spongiform appearance of the
right ventricle to make this diagnosis. In these cases, trabeculations are seen in
the lateral wall of the right ventricle with hyper-trabeculation up to the tricuspid
valve, particularly in severe cases [3]. The implications of biventricular involvement remain unknown [7–9, 57–59].

8. *NCCM with Congenital Heart Disease*: NCCM has been reported in association
with most all congenital heart lesions and may contribute to myocardial dysfunction and/or arrhythmias. Right-sided lesions, especially Ebstein's anomaly, pulmonic stenosis, pulmonary atresia, tricuspid atresia, and double outlet right

ventricle, are most common with septal defects and left heart defects less commonly seen [10, 23, 26–29, 60]. Outcomes are dependent on the specific form of congenital heart disease. However, the inclusion of NCCM with congenital heart disease increases the risk postoperatively and, if ventricular dysfunction occurs at any time, the outcomes also suffer.

Imaging of Noncompaction Cardiomyopathy in the Childhood

The diagnosis of NCCM relies on non-invasive imaging studies, most typically transthoracic echocardiography and cardiac magnetic resonance imaging (CMR), However, controversy exists regarding the diagnostic criteria used for both modalities. Transthoracic echocardiography remains the most common approach to the diagnosis of NCCM. This is in large part due to widespread availability, interpretability, and cost. The most common criteria for diagnosis uses a ratio of the thickness of the noncompacted layer to the thickness of the compacted layer (T/C) with a ratio >2 at end diastole being considered diagnostic [61]. Alternative diagnostic criteria have been proposed, including T/C ratios ranging between 2:1 and 3:1, but all require expert assessment to discern between normal variants and NCCM [2, 13, 62]. One issue that is perplexing is the use of any ratio of non-compact to compact layer thickness or trabecular length. A reasonable question is why would the size of trabeculations or ration of layer thicknesses matter? Another possibility would be that the position of the trabeculations and the density of trabeculations are critical for diagnosis. Some data exists regarding these diagnostic quandaries. Punn and Silverman performed a retrospective analysis of children with NCCM using the 16-segment model described by the American Heart Association and the American Society of Echocardiography [63]. Left ventricular ejection fraction was inversely related to the number of segments involved and, in younger patients, poor outcomes as defined by death or transplantation were related to the number of segments affected. Advanced echocardiographic techniques such as strain, strain rate, and torsion are now being used as well to assist in the diagnosis of NCCM [64–66]. Authors supporting the ratios of layers support their viewpoints using statistical evidence; however, no gold standard exists to compare this data against. However, due to the lack of definitive diagnostic criteria, concerns have been raised that NCCM has gone from being under-recognized to being over-diagnosed.

Cardiac MRI is becoming increasingly used in the diagnosis and ongoing surveillance of NCCM in both children and adults and the same controversies exist as described for echocardiography (Fig. 7.3). The diagnostic criteria for the NCCM are also based on the T/C ratio, with a ratio >2.3 at end diastole typically used [67]. However, as with echocardiography, there is a lack of consensus regarding this definition. Thuny et al. [68] evaluated 16 patients with NCCM who underwent both echocardiography and CMR within the same week for comparison. They utilized a standard 17-segment anatomical model and found that the extent of NCCM was better defined by CMR and that CMR also provided additional morphological characterization of the myocardium. Jacquier et al. [69] proposed diagnostic CMR

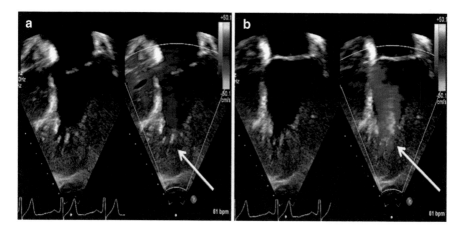

Fig. 7.3 Diagnosis of left ventricular noncompaction. Color Doppler transthoracic echocardiogram four chamber view zoomed in at the hyper-trabeculated left ventricle with color flow (**a**) in (red) and (**b**) out (blue) of intra-trabecular recesses (white arrows)

criteria that assess the amount of left ventricular mass and burden of trabeculations, with trabeculations >20% of the total mass being diagnostic. Cardiac MRI also offers the opportunity to assess for myocardial fibrosis with the presence of delayed/late gadolinium enhancement (LGE) possibly offering prognostic information [70, 71]. Also notable, CMR has shown that the compact layer is commonly abnormally thin, especially at the apex, and can actually be confused with being an apical aneurysm. More recently, cardiac computed tomography has been used and is capable of showing the abnormal architecture of the left ventricular wall in noncompaction. Cardiac computed tomography (CCT) enables quantitative and qualitative assessment of global and regional ventricular function, and is excellent to exclude coronary artery disease or anomalies, which is usually not feasible with CMR or echocardiography [72]. Since CT is associated with very high radiation doses, while echocardiography and CMR has no radiation exposure, this is an important and limiting concern due to its oncologic potential especially in children or in patients requiring long-term, repeated surveillance [73].

Our group uses a matrix of data to make the diagnosis of NCCM. The criteria used for transthoracic echocardiography includes a combination of location of trabeculations, density of trabeculations, and visualization of blood flow into the intertrabecular recesses by color Doppler interrogation on apical four-chamber view. In addition, we measure the T/C ratio for completeness as well as evaluating the thickness of the compact layer compared to normal. We also use the parasternal short axis view to trigger suspicion of the potential diagnosis, facilitating a higher likelihood that attention will be paid to this possible diagnosis. We use a similar approach for CMR but also use gadolinium to evaluate for scar burden. In addition, we carefully evaluate left ventricular size, thickness, systolic function and diastolic function, atrial size and volume, as well as analyzing for any associated congenital heart defects. Finally, a careful analysis of the right ventricle and its trabeculation-burden should be evaluated.

An extensive revision of the diagnostic challenges and the current literature is described in the Chap. 3 of this book by Soliman et al.

Electrocardiography (ECG) in Noncompaction Cardiomyopathy

The ECG in patients with NCCM is typically abnormal; in up to 87% of patient's ECG findings of hypertrophy by voltage criteria (either left ventricular hypertrophy or biventricular hypertrophy), T wave inversion, ST segment abnormalities or strain, left atrial enlargement, left axis deviation, QTc prolongation, or pre-excitation will be seen (Figs. 7.4 and 7.5). In neonates and young children, extreme QRS voltages may be seen [3, 14, 50, 53, 74].

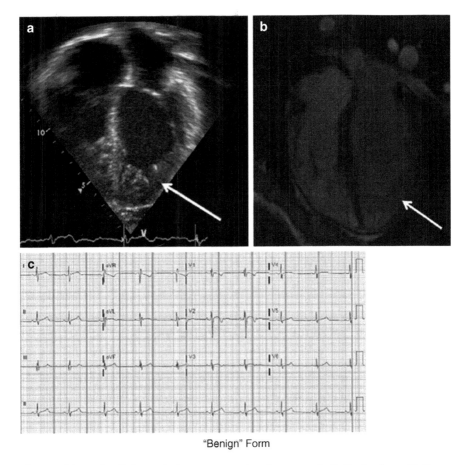

"Benign" Form

Fig. 7.4 Diagnosis of left ventricular noncompaction phenotypes. Left: Benign form of left ventricular noncompaction in a 15 year old male. (**a**) Transthoracic echocardiogram and (**b**) cardiac MRI four chamber views with trabeculations and intra-trabecular recesses (white arrows) at the apex and apical lateral wall; (**c**) Twelve lead electrocardiogram with normal sinus rhythm, low QRS voltages, and interventricular conduction delay

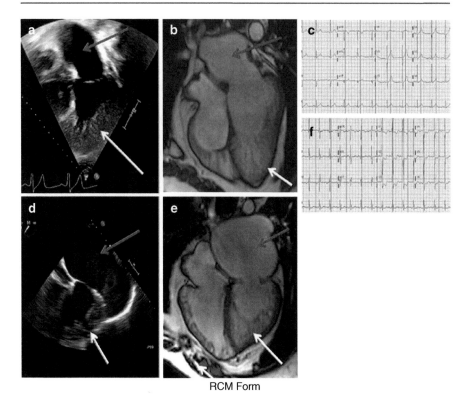

RCM Form

Fig. 7.5 Right: Restrictive cardiomyopathy form of left ventricular noncompaction. (**a**) Transthoracic echocardiogram and (**b**) cardiac MRI four chamber views in a 44 year old male with trabeculations (white arrows) in all apical wall segments and severe left atrial dilation (red arrows), and (**c**) 12 lead electrocardiogram with normal sinus rhythm and left ventricular hypertrophy; (**d**) transesophageal echocardiogram and (**e**) cardiac MRI four chamber views in a 20 year old female with trabeculations (white arrows) in all apical wall segments and severe left atrial dilation (red arrows), and (**f**) 12 lead electrocardiogram with low right atrial rhythm, biventricular hypertrophy with ST segment depression in the precordial leads

Arrhythmias in Noncompaction Cardiomyopathy

Supraventricular and ventricular arrhythmias, as well as bradyarrhythmias are frequently observed in NCCM, with many being life-threatening [50]. As noted previously, the NCCM sub-type that presents with early-onset rhythm abnormalities generally has significant risk of sudden death. Implantable cardioverter defibrillators (ICDs) have been shown to be highly effective for the prevention of sudden arrhythmic death in NCCM patients, including patients with severe left ventricular dysfunction, a prior history of sustained ventricular tachycardia or ventricular fibrillation, recurrent syncope of unknown etiology, or a family history of sudden cardiac death. Ventricular tachyarrhythmias, including those seen in subjects having cardiac arrest due to ventricular fibrillation, has been reported in 38–47% of adult patients with NCCM and in 13–18% of subjects experiencing sudden death [18, 28, 29, 41, 43]. Caliskan et al. [75] investigated the indications and outcomes of ICD therapy in 77 adult NCCM patients, 57% of whom had an ICD implanted using standard implant guidelines for non-ischemic cardiomyopathy. During a mean follow-up of 33 ± 24 months, eight patients presented with appropriate defibrillator shocks due to sustained ventricular tachycardia after a median of 6.1 (1–16) months, suggesting that NCCM patients could be at high risk for sudden cardiac death. All of the appropriate defibrillator interventions in this patient cohort were due to fast ventricular tachycardias, although it is not certain that the initial rhythm in those patients suffering sudden cardiac death due to ventricular fibrillation was also initiated by a ventricular tachycardia trigger. In NCCM patients presenting with sustained ventricular arrhythmias, there was a 33% risk of recurrent sustained ventricular tachycardia followed by appropriate defibrillator shocks after a median follow-up period of 26 months. Similarly, Kobza et al. reported appropriate shocks in 37% of patients with NCCM and an ICD at a mean follow-up of 40 months [76]. In small children, pharmacologic anti-arrhythmia therapies may be indicated prior to consideration of an implantable cardioverter defibrillator due to the high rate of lead fractures and inappropriate shocks in this population. In addition, Van Malderen et al. evaluated 101 patients with NCCM to determine the origin of premature ventricular contractions (PVCs) in NCCM and to identify any predominant arrhythmic foci [77]. A total number of 2069 electrocardiograms were studied to determine the origin of PVCs and echocardiographic data were analyzed in patients with PVCs in all 12 leads. Segments affected by NCCM were compared with the origin of PVCs. PVCs were documented in 250 ECGs from 55 (54%) patients. Thirty-five ECGs recorded PVCs on all 12 leads and the origin of 20 types of PVCs could be determined. Ninety-five percent of PVCs did not originate from left ventricular noncompact myocardial areas and two PVCs (10%) had a true myocardial origin. All other PVCs originated from structures such as the outflow tracts (8/20), the fascicles (7/20), especially the posteromedial fascicle (6/20), and the mitral and tricuspid annulus (3/20), suggesting that PVCs in NCCM mainly originate from the conduction system and related myocardium (Figs. 7.6 and 7.7).

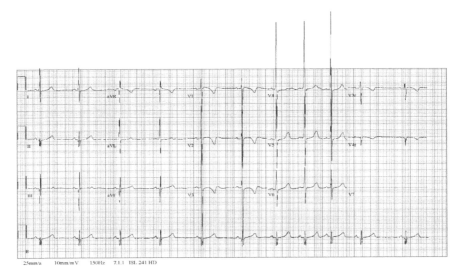

Fig. 7.6 Electrocardiogram diagnosis of left ventricular noncompaction. Electrocardiogram from a 17 year old patient with NCCM in whom prominent precordial voltage is notable

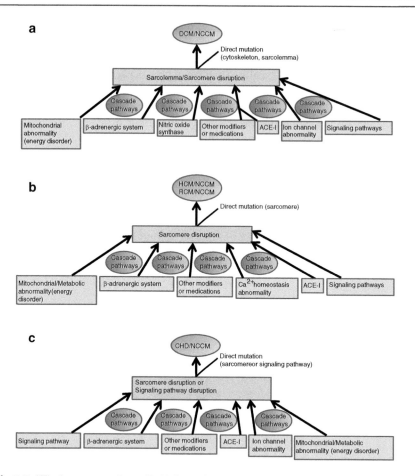

Fig. 7.7 "Final common pathways" of left ventricular noncompaction. (**a**) Dilated cardiomyopathy occurs due to either direct mutation, most typically in sarcomere protein- or cytoskeletal protein-encoding genes, or secondary disruption of the sarcomere-sarcolemmal link through "cascade pathways", including energy production or utilization abnormalities caused by mitochondrial or other metabolic pathway dysfunction, β-adrenergic nervous system dysfunction, or abnormalities in nitric oxide synthase, modifiers (genetic, protein, medications, etc.), angiotensin-converting enzyme inhibitor isoforms, ion channel dysfunction, or signaling pathway disturbance; (**b**) Final common pathways of the hypertrophic or restrictive cardiomyopathy forms of LV noncompaction. Hypertrophic or restrictive cardiomyopathy forms of LV noncompaction occur due to disruption of sarcomere function that result in structural myocardial abnormalities either via direct mutation in sarcomere protein-encoding genes, or secondary disruption of sarcomere function through "cascade pathways", including energy production or utilization abnormalities caused by mitochondrial or other metabolic pathway disturbance, β-adrenergic nervous system dysfunction, modifiers (genetic, protein, medications, etc.), calcium homeostasis abnormalities, angiotensin-converting enzyme inhibitor isoforms, or signaling pathway disturbance; (**c**) Final common pathways of the congenital heart disease form of LV noncompaction. LV noncompaction with congenital heart disease occurs due to disruption of overlapping pathways that result in structural myocardial abnormalities and in developmental pathways, either direct mutation, most typically in sarcomere protein-encoding genes or developmental signaling pathway genes, or secondary disruption of sarcomere or signaling pathway function through "cascade pathways", including signaling pathway disruption, β-adrenergic nervous system dysfunction, modifiers (genetic, protein, medications, etc.), angiotensin-converting enzyme inhibitor isoforms, ion channel dysfunction, or energy production or utilization abnormalities caused by disturbance of mitochondrial or other metabolic pathways

Outcomes Based on Phenotype

The National Heart, Lung, and Blood Institute-funded Pediatric Cardiomyopathy Registry reported on 3219 children with cardiomyopathy, identifying 155 children (4.8%) with definitive NCCM diagnosed from 1990 to 2008 [78]. Each child diagnosed with NCCM patient was classified as having an associated echocardiographically diagnosed cardiomyopathy phenotype including dilated, hypertrophic, restrictive, isolated, or indeterminate. They observed a significant difference among the phenotypic groups in time to death or transplant with isolated NCCM having the best outcomes, followed by those with the HCM-form of NCCM. Children with the DCM-form of NCCM and the indeterminate cardiomyopathy phenotype had the worst outcomes. The hazard ratio for death/transplant (with isolated NCCM as the reference group) was 4.26 (95% confidence interval [CI], 0.78–23.3) for the HCM-form of NCCM, 6.35 (95% CI, 1.52–26.6) for the DCM-form of NCCM, and 5.66 (95% CI, 1.04–30.9) for the indeterminate phenotype. Time to listing for cardiac transplantation significantly differed by phenotype ($P < 0.001$), as did time to transplantation ($P = 0.015$). Five-year transplant rates were 0% for isolated NCCM or the HCM-form of NCCM, 27% for the DCM-form of NCCM, and 27% for the indeterminate phenotype group. Five-year rates for the combined endpoint of death or transplant (and death or listing) were 33% (35%) for the entire NCCM cohort; phenotype specific rates were 6% (6%) of isolated NCCM, 43% (45%) for the DCM-form of NCCM, 25% (25%) for the HCM-form of NCCM, and 33% (42%) for the indeterminate phenotype groups.

Very few isolated NCCM patients developed an associated cardiomyopathy phenotype. Of the 35 cases with isolated NCCM, the 2 deaths observed occurred shortly after diagnosis. One of the deceased patients had an associated DCM phenotype on repeat echocardiogram. Of the remaining 33 isolated NCCM cases, a 2-year repeat echocardiogram was available in 24 subjects, with two showing characteristics of HCM. Therefore, they estimated that 12% (3 of 25) progressed to an associated cardiomyopathy phenotype within 2 years. One additional case was reported as RCM at 1 year but this was done without an associated supporting echocardiogram. This patient was alive at 4 years with an LV wall thickness Z score of <-2, normal LV systolic function, and no evidence of an associated RM phenotype by echocardiogram at that time. The authors concluded that the specific NCCM-associated cardiomyopathy phenotype predicts the risk of death or transplantation and should inform clinical management.

van Waning et al. [79] studied a cohort of 52 children and adults. Eighty-three percent of the children and 85% of the adults were symptomatic at presentation. Heart failure (27%) and arrhythmias (26%) were the most common presentations in children and adults. In 4%, the primary presentation was cardiac arrest. Thromboembolic events were the first sign of NCCM in 3%, with stroke seen in 70% of these individuals. Major adverse cardiac events were relatively common, with 27% of children, and 21% of adults experiencing major adverse cardiac events during a median follow-up of 25 months.

Clinical Genetics of Noncompaction Cardiomyopathy

NCCM has been identified in families with X-linked inheritance, autosomal dominant and autosomal recessive inheritance, as well as maternally inherited (matrilin-
ear) mitochondrial inheritance [3, 10, 30, 80]. In addition, sporadic cases are
common, probably involved in 60–70% of cases. Although several NCCM-
susceptibility genes have been identified to date, none predominate, and systematic
evaluations of large populations have not been reported. NCCM arising from these
genetic causes are associated typically with rare non-synonymous variants, primarily missense, with occasional nonsense, splice site or small insertion/deletion variants. More than any other form of cardiomyopathy, mitochondrial disease is a
prominent feature of infants and young children with NCCM and therefore requires
evaluation [30]. When NCCM is associated with congenital heart disease, the congenital cardiac defect may be heterogeneous in families but this form of NCCM is
transmitted as an autosomal dominant trait along with the congenital heart abnormality [10]. In some families with autosomal dominant NCCM associated with congenital heart disease, affected members may be identified in whom no congenital
heart disease can be identified at the time of initial evaluation because the cardiac
defects include "minor" forms of disease (e.g., small ventricular and atrial septal
defects, or patent ductus arteriosus), which have spontaneously closed, while other
family members have severe forms of congenital heart disease (e.g., hypoplastic left
heart syndrome, Ebstein's anomaly, etc.) [28, 29, 60]. Penetrance may be reduced in
some families. Ichida et al. [14] reported that 44% of her NCCM patients had inherited NCCM, with 70% having autosomal dominant and 30% X-linked inheritance.
As noted, chromosomal abnormalities and syndromic patients also have been identified with NCCM [81]. Digilio et al. investigated the prevalence of chromosomal
abnormalities in 25 syndromic patients with NCCM using standard cytogenetic,
sub-telomeric fluorescent in situ hybridization (FISH), and array-CGH analysis.
Standard chromosome analysis was abnormal in 3 (12%) patients (45,X/46,XX
mosaic, 45,X/46,X,i(Y)(p11) mosaic, and de novo Robertsonian 13;14 transloca-
tion) while cryptic chromosome anomalies were found in 6 (24%) cases (1p36 deletion, 7p14.3p14.1 deletion, 18p sub-telomeric deletion, 22q11.2 deletion, and distal
22q11.2 deletion) [81]. NCCM and trisomy 18 and with trisomy 13 have also been
described [82, 83]. NCCM has also been associated with chromosome 8p23.1 deletion [84]. Other syndromes associated with NCCM include Coffin-Lowry syndrome, caused by mutations in the RPS6KA3 gene on chromosome Xp22.2,
encoding the ribosomal protein S6 kinase-2 (RSK2) [85], and Sotos syndrome, due
to mutations in the nuclear receptor binding SET domain protein 1 (NSD1) gene on
chromosome 5q35, encoding a histone methyltransferase implicated in transcrip-
tional regulation via chromatin remodeling [86, 87]. Sellars et al. described a newborn with tetrasomy 5q35.2-5q35.3 having NCCM and absent thumbs, possibly
consistent with an association with Hunter-McAlpine syndrome [88], while Corrado
et al. reported NCCM and Charcot-Marie-Tooth disease type 1A from duplication
in PMP22 [89].

Index Cases

A relatively small percentage of patients with NCCM have known genetic mutations, probably on the order of 20–30%, though larger panels of genes can increase the yield proportionately. For instance, Klassen and colleagues reported a 17% rate of mutation detection when looking at six genes among 63 unrelated adult probands [90]. Hoedemaekers et al. reported use of a 17-gene panel in which mutations were recognized in 23 of 56 probands (41%) [91]. The clinical diagnosis of NCCM depends on particular expertise and knowledge of disease and imaging modalities, particularly echocardiography and cardiac magnetic resonance imaging (CMR), and is supported by electrocardiographic findings. Due to the low rate of a positive genetic test in index cases to date, the authors suggested that the utility of genetic testing for the definitive diagnosis and care of the index case is currently of limited use. More recently, van Waning et al. [79] reported on 327 unrelated patients (primarily adults) with NCCM, with 52 of these patients being children. In this group, 40% were sporadic presentations, with 60% being familial of which 45% were genetic with mutations identified, and 15% were probably genetic but no mutations were identified. The mutations noted in these children were mostly in sarcomere-encoding genes (*MYH7* in 19%, *MYBPC3* in 8%, other sarcomere-encoding genes in 6%, and non-sarcomeric genes in 12%). In the adult cohort, 40% were familial with only 30% having mutations, including mutations mostly in sarcomere-encoding genes (*MYH7* in 11%, *TTN* in 7%, *MYBPC3* in 4%, other sarcomere-encoding genes in 3%, and non-sarcomeric genes in 5%).

Family Relatives

Identification of a definite pathogenic mutation in clinically affected probands should lead to screening of all at-risk (siblings, parents, children) including those individuals with a negative phenotype. One of the important aspects of genetic testing is the ability to confirm mutation-positive or mutation-negative status in family members of clinically affected, genotype-positive subjects. Due to possible X-linked inheritance in some patients, affected male family members may have a pronounced disease expression and females may have milder signs of NCCM (or none at all) and, thus, may serve as transmitters for following generations. Somatic mitochondrial alterations are, in general, not heritable to next generations and require a different clinical and genetic consultation.

Prognostic Role of Genetic Testing for NCCM

No genotype-phenotype correlations have been associated with NCCM to date and therefore no prognostic implications can be speculated. The only implication of genetic testing at present is confirmation of diagnosis and the potential development of disease in mutation-positive members of the family, if tested. Therapy, therefore, is completely based on phenotypic findings. Miller et al. [92] recently reported genetic testing on 75 children with NCCM, of which 59% were idiopathic, 32% had familial disease, and 9% had a syndromic or metabolic diagnosis. In 65 individuals, a cardiomyopathy gene panel was performed and the other ten patients had known variant testing performed. The yield of cardiomyopathy gene panel testing was 9%. The severity of NCCM by imaging criteria was not associated with positive genetic testing, co-occurring cardiac features, pathogenesis, family history, or myocardial dysfunction. Individuals with isolated NCCM were significantly less likely to have a positive genetic testing result compared with those with NCCM associated with an overlapping form of cardiomyopathy (0% versus 12%, respectively). The authors suggested that genetic testing should be considered in individuals with NCCM associated with an overlapping form of cardiomyopathy but cardiomyopathy gene panel testing in individuals with isolated NCCM in the absence of a family history of cardiomyopathy was probably not indicated.

Therapeutic Role of Genetic Testing for NCCM

No definitive therapeutic role has been established for NCCM genetic testing. Because associated mitochondrial or metabolic disease (such as Barth syndrome), or syndromes are frequently associated with NCCM, especially in young children, firm diagnosis can lead to improved symptomatic therapy and improved prognostication in affected patients and family members [93, 94]. In addition, identification of mutations in certain genes (such as lamin A/C, SCN5A, HCN4) [95–99] can facilitate assessment of arrhythmias and early treatment with medications or implantable cardioversion defibrillator (ICD).

Molecular Genetics of Noncompaction Cardiomyopathy

The genetic cause of NCCM, like the clinical phenotype itself, is heterogeneous. However, like the genetic causes of other forms of cardiomyopathy, NCCM genetics also follows a "final common pathway" [97, 100]. The specific final common pathway, however, depends on the clinical phenotype and mirrors the genetic causes of the clinical subtype in cardiomyopathies devoid of NCCM. For instance, the "final common pathway" of hypertrophic cardiomyopathy is dysfunction of the sarcomere and, in support of this concept, the vast majority of the genes identified in cases of inherited of hypertrophic cardiomyopathy either encode for sarcomere proteins (such as β-myosin heavy chain) or encode for proteins that disrupt the function of the sarcomere (such as mitochondrial electron transport chain proteins; see below). However, in NCCM, there appears to be a disturbance of more than a single "final common pathway" and, in most cases, probably disturbs a primary pathway (such as the sarcomere) and a developmental pathway (such as the NOTCH pathway; see section on Animal Models of NCCM, below), commonly via a disturbance of protein-protein binding caused by the primary genetic mutation.

The first genetic cause of NCCM without evidence of congenital heart disease was initially described by Bleyl et al. [101] who identified mutations in the X-linked TAZ gene in patients and carrier females. TAZ encodes the tafazzin protein, a phospholipid transacylase that is important for membrane function and, when mutated typically causes the multisystem human disorder called Barth syndrome, which is characterized by cardiomyopathy (commonly NCCM), skeletal myopathy, cyclic neutropenia, 3-methylglutaconic aciduria (a marker of mitochondrial dysfunction), and deficiency of a key membrane phospholipid of cardiomyocytes and mitochondria called cardiolipin. It is believed that this defect disturbs mitochondrial function, leading to a combination of an energy production-energy utilization abnormality and, because the sarcomere requires energy in the form of adenosine triphosphate (ATP), sarcomere dysfunction (see section on Animal Models of NCCM, below).

Multiple genes causing autosomal dominant NCCM have since been identified, including mutations in genes causing congenital heart disease with NCCM. Mutations in ~20 genes have been implicated and mostly include cytoskeletal, sarcomeric, and ion channel genes, with sarcomere-encoding genes being most common. In addition, syndromal disorders such as Barth syndrome and muscular dystrophies are known to be associated with NCCM as well. In patients with hypoplastic left heart syndrome and NCCM, we identified α-dystrobrevin causative mutations while mutations in Nkx-2.5 was identified in children with NCCM and atrial septal defect and both β-myosin heavy chain (MYH7) mutations and α-tropomyosin (TPM1) have been reported in patients with NCCM and Ebstein's anomaly [102–104].

The most common genes identified include the sarcomere-encoding genes β-myosin heavy chain (*MYH7*), α-cardiac actin (*ACTC1*), cardiac troponin T (*TNNT2*), myosin binding protein-C (MYBPC3) and *ZASP* (*also called LIM-domain binding protein 3, LBD3*) [91, 104–106]. In addition, mutations in α-tropomyosin (TPM1) and cardiac troponin I (TNNI3) also have been identified. Hoedemaekers et al. [91] additionally demonstrated an association of NCCM with genetic variants in two calcium handling genes, as well as TAZ and lamin A/C (LMNA). Probst et al. [105] further showed that sarcomere gene mutations are important in NCCM, showing a prevalence of 29%, with MYH7 and MYBPC3 most frequently mutated (13% and 8%, respectively). Dellefave et al. [106] also identified sarcomere mutations in NCCM, including those presenting with heart failure in infancy. Recently, Hasdtings et al. performed whole genome sequencing, linkage analysis, and functional studies on two families with NCCM and identified missense mutations in titin (TTN), which encodes the giant titin protein found in the Z-disk and sarcomere [107]. Bagnall and colleagues showed an association of NCCM, idiopathic ventricular fibrillation, and sudden death with a mutation in the ACTN2 gene in a family [108]. van Waning et al. [79] reported 104 genetic cases with mutations, and 82% involved a sarcomere gene. In most of these cases (71%), a mutation was identified in *MYH7, MYBPC3*, or *TTN*, and 11% had a mutation in *ACTC1, ACTN2, MYL2, TNNC1, TNNT2*, or *TPM1*. In children, no *TTN* mutations were noted. These authors also identified mutations in the non-sarcomere encoding genes DES, DSP, FKTN, HCN4, KCNQ1, LAMP2, *LMNA*, MIB1, NOTCH1, PLN, RYR2, SCN5A, and *TAZ*.

In addition to sarcomere-encoding and cytoskeleton-encoding genes, we demonstrated that mutations in the sodium channel gene (SCN5A) are associated with NCCM and rhythm disturbance [96]. Another cytoskeletal protein associated with NCCM is dystrophin, the gene causing Duchenne and B ecker muscular dystrophy in boys [109]. In addition, homozygous deletions in desmoplakin (DSP) and plakophillin 2 (PKP2), desmosomal protein-encoding genes known to cause arrhythmogenic cardiomyopathy and dilated cardiomyopathy, have also been identified in NCCM patients [58, 110]. Mitochondrial genome mutations have also been identified to be associated with NCCM [111] and, as noted, chromosomal abnormalities and syndromic patients also have been identified with NCCM [3, 81] including 1p36 deletion, 7p14.3p14.1 deletion, 18p subtelomeric deletion, 22q11.2 deletion, distal 22q11.2, trisomies 18 and 13, 8p23.1 deletion, tetrasomy 5q35.2-5q35, Coffin-Lowry syndrome (RPS6KA3 mutation), Sotos syndrome (NSD1 mutation), and Charcot-Marie-Tooth disease type 1A (PMP22 duplication) [81–89, 112, 113].

Diagnostic testing in patients with NCCM appear to have a detection rate of clinically significant variants in 35–40% of individuals, with sarcomere-encoding genes most commonly found to be mutated [114].

Animal Models of NCCM

A number of mouse models with NCCM have been described over the past several years. These models are being used to discern the underlying mechanism(s) of this form of cardiomyopathy. The most common conclusion reached to date from these studies is that hyper-trabeculation results from altered regulation in cell proliferation, differentiation, and maturation during ventricular wall formation, particularly if the NOTCH signaling pathway is altered. Other hypotheses also exist based on some of the models described below.

FKBP12 Null Mutation FKBP12, also known as Fkbp1a, is a member of the immunophilin protein family that interacts with multiple intracellular protein complexes such as calcium release channels (inositol triphosphate receptor and ryanodine receptor), BMP/activin/TGFβ type-1 receptors, voltage-gated Na^+ channels, FK506 and rapamycin, and inhibits calcineurin and mTOR activity [115–118]. FKBP12-deficient mice develop ventricular hyper-trabeculation and noncompaction. Shou et al. reported previously that a mutant mouse model deficient in FKBP12 develop multiple abnormalities in cardiac structure including lack of compaction, thin ventricular wall, deep inter-trabecular recesses, increased trabeculae, and ventricular septal defect [119]. Chen et al. showed FKBP12 to be a novel negative modulator of activated NOTCH1 reporting that overexpression of FKBP12 significantly reduced NOTCH1 stability and direct inhibition of NOTCH signaling significantly reduced hyper-trabeculation in FKBP12-deficient mice [120]. These findings suggested that FKBP12-mediated regulation of NOTCH1 plays an important role in intercellular communication between endocardium and myocardium, which is crucial in controlling the formation of the ventricular walls [116].

MIB1 Mutant Further support for NOTCH1 pathway disturbance as a contributor to NCCM development was shown in families with autosomal dominant NCCM and germline mutations (V943F and R530X) in human MIB1 (mindbomb homolog 1) [121]. MIB1 encodes for an E3 ubiquitin ligase that is involved in regulation of the endocytosis of the NOTCH ligands DELTA and JAGGED. The patients with MIB1 had reduced NOTCH1 activity, Biventricular noncompaction including NCCM with a dilated phenotype, and heart failure. Functional studies in mice targeting MIB1 inactivation in mouse myocardium resulted in NCCM due to arrest of trabecular maturation and ventricular compaction.

Bmp10 Mutant BMP10 is a growth factor that is a member of the TGF-β superfamily that has been shown to be up-regulated in FKBP12 deficient mice [122]. BMP10 is only expressed briefly in the ventricular myocardium during a critical time when development is shifting from patterning to chamber maturation (E9.0 to E13.5) and its ventricular expression is restricted to the trabecular myocardium during this stage. BMP10-deficient mice typically die in utero at around E10.5 with evidence of very hypoplastic ventricular walls without trabeculae [18]. BMP overexpression leads to NCCM and ventricular septal defect. Up-regulation of BMP10 also results in a hyper-trabeculation phenotype in Numb/Numblike-deficient and Nkx2.5-knockout mice (see below) [22, 122, 123]. These findings suggest that BMP10 is an important factor in cardiac trabeculation/compaction.

Tbx20 Mutant Tbx20 is a member of the Tbx1 subfamily of the T-box family transcription factors. Its expression in mouse embryos can be detected in the cardiac precursor cells at E7.5, persists in the developing myocardium and endocardium at E8.0, and at later developmental stages its expression is more abundant in the atrium compared with the ventricles. In addition, Tbx20 is a key mediator of BMP10 signaling in ventricular wall development and maturation [35]. Over-expression of Tbx20 led to a severe dilated cardiomyopathy with hyper-trabeculation consistent with the dilated cardiomyopathy form of NCCM [35].

Numb/Numb-Like Mutant Numb family proteins, including Numb and numblike, are cell fate determinants for multiple progenitor cell types (hematopoietic stem cells, muscle satellite cells, cancer stem cells, and hemangioblasts), doing so by maintaining neural stem cell fate and regulating its differentiation. In addition, Numb functions as a component of the adherens junction to regulate cell adhesion and migration, complexes with β-catenin to regulate Wnt signaling, and interacts with integrin β subunits to promote their endocytosis for directional cell migration. When Numb and Numb-like are deleted in mouse hearts by Nkx2.5[Cre/], creating a myocardial double knockout of these two genes, NCCM with congenital heart disease occurs [22, 123]. The congenital heart defects include atrioventricular septal defects, truncus arteriosus, and double outlet right ventricle. This model demonstrates that Numb family proteins regulate trabecular thickness by inhibiting Notch1 signaling, control cardiac morphogenesis in a Notch1-independent manner, and regulate cardiac progenitor cell differentiation in an endocytosis-dependent manner.

Nkx2-5 Mutant Mice that harbor a ventricular muscle cell-restricted knockout of Nkx2-5 develop progressive atrioventricular block with progressive conduction system cell dropout and fibrosis with NCCM also being a prominent feature in neonatal mice, with progressive biventricular dilation and heart failure developing early [124]. Nkx2-5, a cardiac homeobox gene, is a transcription factor that regulates heart development in humans, working along with MEF2, HAND1, and HAND2 transcription factors to direct heart looping during early heart development. NKX 2-5 directly activates the MEF2 gene to control cardiomyocyte differentiation and operates in a positive feedback loop with GATA transcription factors to regulate cardiomyocyte formation. Ashraf et al. generated a murine model in a 129/Sv genetic background by knocking-in an Nkx2-5 homeodomain missense mutation previously identified in human, as missense mutations in the NKX2-5 homeodomain (DNA-binding domain) are the most frequently reported type of human mutation [125]. All heterozygous neonatal Nkx2-5(+/R52G) mice demonstrated a prominent trabecular layer in the ventricular wall along with diverse cardiac anomalies, including atrioventricular septal defects, Ebstein malformation of the tricuspid valve, and perimembranous and muscular ventricular septal defects. These results suggest that heterozygous missense mutation in the murine Nkx2-5 homeodomain (R52G) is highly penetrant and results in pleiotropic cardiac effects. In contrast to heterozygous Nkx2-5 knockout mice, the effects of the heterozygous knockin mice mimic findings in humans with heterozygous missense mutation in NKX2-5 homeodomain. Heterozygous human mutations of NKX2-5 are highly penetrant and associated with varied congenital heart defects. The heterozygous knockout of murine Nkx2-5, in contrast, manifests less profound cardiac malformations, with low disease penetrance.

Smad7 Mutant TGF-β superfamily members exert their biological functions by binding to serine/threonine kinase receptors at the cell surface, followed by signal transduction by the intracellular transducers called Smads [126, 127]. Smad proteins can be classified into three functional subclasses, with Smad7 being an inhibitory Smad. Smad7-deficient mutant mice typically die in utero due to multiple defects in cardiovascular development, including ventricular septal defect and NCCM, as well as outflow tract malformations and heart failure [126]. When Smad7 mutant mice live to adulthood, NCCM with impaired cardiac function and severe arrhythmia is notable.

NF-ATc Mutant The expression of early response genes in lymphocytes is regulated by NF-AT transcription factors. NF-ATc mutant embryos have multiple cardiac abnormalities including myocardial developmental abnormalities, narrowing or occlusion of the ventricular outflow tract, defective septum morphogenesis, and underdevelopment of the semilunar valves with half of the mice dying at day E14.5 from circulatory failure [128]. In 40% of the mutant embryos, ventricular hypertrophy and small chamber size is seen as well as NCCM with hyper-trabeculation commonly seen, suggesting that NF-AT signaling pathways are important for valve and septum development as well as development of hyper-trabeculation/ noncompaction.

Jarid2/Jumonji Mutants The Jumonji family proteins function as histone demethylases [129]. Jarid2/Jumonji critically regulates developmental processes including cardiovascular development, as demonstrated by Jarid2 knock-out mice which have LV noncompaction associated with a thin compact layer, ventricular septal defects and double outlet right ventricle [130–132]. Mysliwiec et al. [132] showed that the NOTCH1 pathway is directly controlled by Jarid2 and that failure to regulate NOTCH1 expression, as is the case in Jarid2 knockout mice, leads to proliferation and differentiation defects in the developing heart which are manifested in the form of LV noncompaction associated with a thin ventricular wall. Deletion of NOTCH1 in the mouse has also been shown to result in impaired trabeculation and myocardial proliferation associated with embryonic lethality due to cardiac insufficiency [133].

Tafazzin (TAZ) Mutant Barth syndrome, an X-linked, multisystem human disorder characterized by cardiomyopathy (commonly NCCM), skeletal myopathy, cyclic neutropenia, 3-methylglutaconic aciduria, and cardiolipin deficiency, a key membrane phospholipid of cardiomyocytes and mitochondria, is caused by mutations in the X-linked gene tafazzin (TAZ) [10, 23, 134]. A TAZ knockdown mouse model has been shown to develop NCCM associated with abnormal cardiolipin profiles and mitochondrial structural abnormalities, indicating that mitochondrial function is important for proper myocardial development [135].

Therapy and Outcome

Therapy in NCCM is predicated on making the correct phenotypic diagnosis given that associated phenotypes require different surveillance and are associated with variable outcomes [5, 10, 14, 27, 50, 100]. Increasing awareness of the disease is resulting in larger numbers of diagnoses. Furthermore, given the heritability of this disease, at-risk first degree relatives are recommended for screening resulting in patients being diagnosed that otherwise would have never undergone noninvasive imaging. The role of clinically available genetic testing has also impacted management. Panels that assess for known sarcomeric gene mutations implicated in NCCM are becoming more commonly used and are considered standard of care in many institutions. In those patients with identified pathologic mutation, targeted sequencing can then be performed on first degree relatives. This has important implications as these sarcomeric genes are known to present as varying cardiac phenotypes within families meaning that a first degree relative of a known NCCM patient harboring the identical mutation may have an NCCM phenotype or instead have isolated dilated, hypertrophic, or restrictive cardiomyopathy without NCCM. These family members could also have the same mutation as the affected individual and have no phenotype at all. The presence of a pathologic mutation alters ongoing screening recommendations and should result in genetic counseling regarding risk to future offspring.

Therapy for NCCM is largely dictated by concomitant clinical findings associated with myocardial dysfunction and/or significant arrhythmias, or congenital heart disease. Patients with evidence of systolic or diastolic dysfunction should be managed based on existing recommendations [136]. For patients with NCCM and associated systolic dysfunction or dilated cardiomyopathy phenotype, oral therapies typically include anti-congestive medications that help to favorably remodel the left ventricle, including angiotensin converting enzyme (ACE) inhibitors and beta blockers, and an aldosterone antagonist. The use of loop diuretics would be considered for patients with evidence of congestion or volume overload and aspirin is used in order to reduce the potential for thrombotic complications. Inpatient therapies may consist of intravenous diuretics and/or vasodilatory agents in the setting of acute decompensated heart failure. Inotropes may be used in patients with evidence of low cardiac output and poor end organ perfusion. Patients may be considered for implantable-cardioverter defibrillators if they meet criteria for implantation as recommended in published guidelines. Advanced pacing strategies such as cardiac resynchronization may also be employed with improvement being seen in some patients [75, 76]. The use of ventricular assist devices and cardiac transplant may also be considered for those patients with end-stage disease. Patients with associated hypertrophic cardiomyopathy may benefit from symptomatic therapies if left ventricular outflow tract obstruction is present in the form of beta blockers or calcium channel blockers. Internal cardioverter-defibrillator placement may be considered for those patients with increased risk of sudden cardiac death [137].

There are well known thromboembolic risks associated with NCCM [14, 138] although these are largely reported in adults [138]. For this reason, treatment with antiplatelet or systemic anticoagulation may be considered in adults, especially when the left ventricle or atria are dilated. The incidence of stroke or other embolic phenomena in children remains poorly characterized. Antiplatelet therapy may be considered in those with depressed left ventricular systolic dysfunction, evidence of spontaneous echocardiographic contrast, severe left ventricular dilation, and/or dilated atria. The presence of atrial fibrillation may also prompt use of systemic anticoagulation.

In patients with primary diastolic dysfunction, pharmacologic therapy may be instituted but no treatments have proven benefit. In many cases, combination systolic and diastolic dysfunction occurs, causing decompensated heart failure requiring the therapeutic approaches noted above. Some patients develop restrictive physiology and these patients generally require transplantation. Management strategies for those patients with the diagnosis of mitochondrial disease or metabolic derangements may be managed with additional medical therapies such as coenzyme Q10, L-carnitine, riboflavin, and thiamine in the setting of known mitochondrial disease. However, the benefit of these therapies is unclear.

In patients with associated congenital heart disease, NCCM may alter therapy and confound outcomes. Treatment of congenital heart disease will be dictated by the severity of the lesion and may require percutaneous or surgical intervention. Furthermore, consideration of overarching genetic causes must be considered which may impact management as well as screening of at-risk family members. The presence of NCCM may complicate management resulting in higher risks of myocardial dysfunction, arrhythmias, and thromboembolic events especially in the perioperative period. Consideration must be given to possible syndromic disease or metabolic diseases, possibly impacting management considerations in patients undergoing catheter-based interventions and/or surgical palliations/corrective surgery. Management will be directed at associated myocardial dysfunction with or without evidence of heart failure as well as significant dysrhythmias.

The outcomes of patients with left ventricular noncompaction are largely associated with the presence of myocardial dysfunction and/or the presence of clinically significant arrhythmias. Brescia et al. [50] reported on our single center experience of 242 children with NCCM. Of these, 150/242 (62%) were noted to have myocardial dysfunction and 80/242 (33.1%) had a significant arrhythmia. The presence of myocardial dysfunction or arrhythmias were strongly associated with mortality (p < 0.001 and p = 0.002. respectively). Similar reports exist in the adult literature citing myocardial dysfunction or ventricular arrhythmias as predictors of mortality.

Conclusions and Summary

Left ventricular noncompaction is a complex, clinically and genetically heterogeneous disorder that with advancement in diagnostic modalities and an increase in awareness has become the third most common cardiomyopathy diagnosed in children and adults. However, controversy remains regarding the diagnostic criteria for NCCM and this area continues to need improvement. NCCM may be associated with congenital heart disease, systemic disorders of metabolism and energy, dysmorphic syndromes, and chromosomal defects. Due to its heterogeneous clinical phenotype, the propensity for the development of associated arrhythmias, sudden cardiac death, and heart failure that is dependent on the specific clinical phenotype, and its current under-recognition by many clinicians, NCCM is a disorder that requires better clinical identification and pathologic understanding in order for improved care and new targeted therapies to be developed and for improved outcomes to continue. In addition, because NCCM overlaps with other forms of cardiomyopathy as well as arrhythmias and congenital heart disease, unraveling the underlying developmental and molecular genetic pathophysiology is likely to enhance our understanding of these other disorders as well, making NCCM a paradigm shifting disorder. The genetic causes are beginning to be determined and understood and animal models are starting to provide insights into the developmental abnormalities that define normal and abnormal development of the compacted and noncompacted myocardium and together these findings may help define the clinical heterogeneity, differential outcomes, and therapies over the next decade.

Recommendations

1. All patients with left ventricular noncompaction should be assessed with at least a three-generation family history, and first-degree relatives should undergo echocardiographic and electrocardiographic testing to determine if their condition is familial.
2. Genetic counseling should be provided to patients with NCCM; this should include discussion of the risks, benefits, and options available for clinical genetic testing.
3. Genetic testing for patients with NCCM can be useful to confirm the diagnosis, to facilitate cascade screening within the family, and to help with family planning.
4. Genetic testing and counseling should be performed in centers experienced in genetic evaluation and family-based management of cardiomyopathy.
5. Patients with NCCM, particularly infants and young children, should be evaluated for metabolic derangements and neuromuscular abnormalities.

Conflicts of Interest The declare that to have no conflicts of interest.

References

1. Grant RT. An unusual anomaly of the coronary vessels in the malformed heart of a child. Heart. 1926;13:273–83.
2. Chin TK, Perloff JK, Williams RG, Jue K, Mohrmann R. Isolated noncompaction of left ventricular myocardium. A study of eight cases. Circulation. 1990;82:507–13.
3. Pignatelli RH, McMahon CJ, Dreyer WJ, et al. Clinical characterization of left ventricular noncompaction in children: a relatively common form of cardiomyopathy. Circulation. 2003;108:2672–8.
4. Engberding R, Yelbuz TM, Breithardt G. Isolated noncompaction of the left ventricular myocardium -- a review of the literature two decades after the initial case description. Clin Res Cardiol. 2007;96:481–8.
5. Sedmera D, Pexieder T, Vuillemin M, Thompson RP, Anderson RH. Developmental patterning of the myocardium. Anat Rec. 2000;258:319–37.
6. Dusek J, Ostadal B, Duskova M. Postnatal persistence of spongy myocardium with embryonic blood supply. Arch Pathol. 1975;99:312–7.
7. Fazio G, Lunetta M, Grassedonio E, et al. Noncompaction of the right ventricle. Pediatr Cardiol. 2010;31:576–8.
8. Ranganathan A, Ganesan G, Sangareddi V, Pillai AP, Ramasamy A. Isolated noncompaction of right ventricle--a case report. Echocardiography. 2012;29:E169–72.
9. Tigen K, Karaahmet T, Gurel E, Cevik C, Basaran Y. Biventricular noncompaction: a case report. Echocardiography. 2008;25:993–6.
10. Towbin JA. Left ventricular noncompaction: a new form of heart failure. Heart Fail Clin. 2010;6:453–69.
11. Maron BJ, Towbin JA, Thiene G, et al. Contemporary definitions and classification of the cardiomyopathies: an American Heart Association Scientific Statement from the Council on Clinical Cardiology, Heart Failure and Transplantation Committee; Quality of Care and Outcomes Research and Functional Genomics and Translational Biology Interdisciplinary Working Groups; and Council on Epidemiology and Prevention. Circulation. 2006;113:1807–16.

12. Stollberger C, Finsterer J, Blazek G. Left ventricular hypertrabeculation/noncompaction and association with additional cardiac abnormalities and neuromuscular disorders. Am J Cardiol. 2002;90:899–902.
13. Stollberger C, Finsterer J. Left ventricular hypertrabeculation/noncompaction. J Am Soc Echocardiogr. 2004;17:91–100.
14. Ichida F, Hamamichi Y, Miyawaki T, et al. Clinical features of isolated noncompaction of the ventricular myocardium: long-term clinical course, hemodynamic properties, and genetic background. J Am Coll Cardiol. 1999;34:233–40.
15. Cartoni D, Salvini P, De Rosa R, Cortese A, Nazzaro MS, Tanzi P. Images in cardiovascular medicine. Multiple coronary artery-left ventricle microfistulae and spongy myocardium: the eagerly awaited link? Circulation. 2007;116:e81–4.
16. Reynen K, Bachmann K, Singer H. Spongy myocardium. Cardiology. 1997;88:601–2.
17. Icardo JM, Fernandez-Teran A. Morphologic study of ventricular trabeculation in the embryonic chick heart. Acta Anat. 1987;130:264–74.
18. Chen H, Zhang W, Li D, Cordes TM, Payne RM, Shou W. Analysis of ventricular hypertrabeculation and noncompaction using genetically engineered mouse models. Pediatr Cardiol. 2009;30:626–34.
19. Harvey RP. Patterning the vertebrate heart. Nat Rev Genet. 2002;3:544–56.
20. Risebro CA, Riley PR. Formation of the ventricles. Sci World J. 2006;6:1862–80.
21. Sedmera D, McQuinn T. Embryogenesis of the heart muscle. Heart Fail Clin. 2008; 4:235–45.
22. Yang J, Bucker S, Jungblut B, et al. Inhibition of Notch2 by Numb/Numblike controls myocardial compaction in the heart. Cardiovasc Res. 2012;96:276–85.
23. Ichida F, Tsubata S, Bowles KR, et al. Novel gene mutations in patients with left ventricular noncompaction or Barth syndrome. Circulation. 2001;103:1256–63.
24. Caliskan K, Ujvari B, Bauernfeind T, et al. The prevalence of early repolarization in patients with noncompaction cardiomyopathy presenting with malignant ventricular arrhythmias. J Cardiovasc Electrophysiol. 2012;23:938–44.
25. Steffel J, Duru F. Rhythm disorders in isolated left ventricular noncompaction. Ann Med. 2012;44:101–8.
26. Attenhofer Jost CH, Connolly HM, Warnes CA, et al. Noncompacted myocardium in Ebstein's anomaly: initial description in three patients. J Am Soc Echocardiogr. 2004;17:677–80.
27. Zuckerman WA, Richmond ME, Singh RK, Carroll SJ, Starc TJ, Addonizio LJ. Left-ventricular noncompaction in a pediatric population: predictors of survival. Pediatr Cardiol. 2011;32:406–12.
28. Stahli BE, Gebhard C, Biaggi P, et al. Left ventricular non-compaction: Prevalence in congenital heart disease. Int J Cardiol. 2013;167:2477–81.
29. Madan S, Mandal S, Bost JE, et al. Noncompaction cardiomyopathy in children with congenital heart disease: evaluation using cardiovascular magnetic resonance imaging. Pediatr Cardiol. 2012;33:215–21.
30. Scaglia F, Towbin JA, Craigen WJ, et al. Clinical spectrum, morbidity, and mortality in 113 pediatric patients with mitochondrial disease. Pediatrics. 2004;114:925–31.
31. Yaplito-Lee J, Weintraub R, Jamsen K, Chow CW, Thorburn DR, Boneh A. Cardiac manifestations in oxidative phosphorylation disorders of childhood. J Pediatr. 2007;150:407–11.
32. Pepper MS. Transforming growth factor-beta: vasculogenesis, angiogenesis, and vessel wall integrity. Cytokine Growth Factor Rev. 1997;8:21–43.
33. Suri C, Jones PF, Patan S, et al. Requisite role of angiopoietin-1, a ligand for the TIE2 receptor, during embryonic angiogenesis. Cell. 1996;87:1171–80.
34. Ferrara N, Carver-Moore K, Chen H, et al. Heterozygous embryonic lethality induced by targeted inactivation of the VEGF gene. Nature. 1996;380:439–42.
35. Zhang W, Chen H, Wang Y, Yong W, Zhu W, Liu Y, Wagner GR, Payne RM, Field LJ, Xin H, Cai CL, Shou W. Tbx20 transcription factor is a downstream mediator for bone morphogenetic protein-10 in regulating cardiac ventricular wall development and function. J Biol Chem. 2011;286(42):36820–9.

36. Stollberger C, Blazek G, Dobias C, Hanafin A, Wegner C, Finsterer J. Frequency of stroke and embolism in left ventricular hypertrabeculation/noncompaction. Am J Cardiol. 2011;108:1021–3.
37. Greutmann M, Mah ML, Silversides CK, et al. Predictors of adverse outcome in adolescents and adults with isolated left ventricular noncompaction. Am J Cardiol. 2012;109:276–81.
38. Steffel J, Kobza R, Oechslin E, Jenni R, Duru F. Electrocardiographic characteristics at initial diagnosis in patients with isolated left ventricular noncompaction. Am J Cardiol. 2009;104:984–9.
39. Celiker A, Ozkutlu S, Dilber E, Karagoz T. Rhythm abnormalities in children with isolated ventricular noncompaction. Pacing Clin Electrophysiol. 2005;28:1198–202.
40. Ritter M, Oechslin E, Sutsch G, Attenhofer C, Schneider J, Jenni R. Isolated noncompaction of the myocardium in adults. Mayo Clin Proc. 1997;72:26–31.
41. Aras D, Tufekcioglu O, Ergun K, et al. Clinical features of isolated ventricular noncompaction in adults long-term clinical course, echocardiographic properties, and predictors of left ventricular failure. J Card Fail. 2006;12:726–33.
42. Sandhu R, Finkelhor RS, Gunawardena DR, Bahler RC. Prevalence and characteristics of left ventricular noncompaction in a community hospital cohort of patients with systolic dysfunction. Echocardiography. 2008;25:8–12.
43. Kovacevic-Preradovic T, Jenni R, Oechslin EN, Noll G, Seifert B, Attenhofer Jost CH. Isolated left ventricular noncompaction as a cause for heart failure and heart transplantation: a single center experience. Cardiology. 2009;112:158–64.
44. Patrianakos AP, Parthenakis FI, Nyktari EG, Vardas PE. Noncompaction myocardium imaging with multiple echocardiographic modalities. Echocardiography. 2008;25:898–900.
45. Ronderos R, Avegliano G, Borelli E, Kuschnir P, Castro F, Sanchez G, Perea G, Corneli M, Zanier MM, Andres S, Aranda A, Conde D, Trivi M. Estimation of prevalence of the left ventricular noncompaction among adults. Am J Cardiol. 2016;118(6):901–5.
46. Sarma RJ, Chana A, Elkayam U. Left ventricular noncompaction. Prog Cardiovasc Dis. 2010;52:264–73.
47. Niemann M, Stork S, Weidemann F. Left ventricular noncompaction cardiomyopathy: an overdiagnosed disease. Circulation. 2012;126:e240-3.
48. Murphy RT, Thaman R, Blanes JG, et al. Natural history and familial characteristics of isolated left ventricular non-compaction. Eur Heart J. 2005;26:187–92.
49. Bhatia NL, Tajik AJ, Wilansky S, Steidley DE, Mookadam F. Isolated noncompaction of the left ventricular myocardium in adults: a systematic overview. J Card Fail. 2011;17:771–8.
50. Brescia ST, Rossano JW, Pignatelli R, et al. Mortality and sudden death in pediatric left ventricular noncompaction in a tertiary referral center. Circulation. 2013;127:2202–8.
51. Caliskan K, Kardos A, Szili-Torok T. Empty handed: a call for an international registry of risk stratification to reduce the 'sudden-ness' of death in patients with non-compaction cardiomyopathy. Europace. 2009;11:1138–9.
52. Biagini E, Ragni L, Ferlito M, et al. Different types of cardiomyopathy associated with isolated ventricular noncompaction. Am J Cardiol. 2006;98:821–4.
53. Ergul Y, Nisli K, Varkal MA, et al. Electrocardiographic findings at initial diagnosis in children with isolated left ventricular noncompaction. Ann Noninvasive Electrocardiol. 2011;16:184–91.
54. Onay OS, Yildirim I, Beken B, et al. Successful implantation of an intracardiac defibrillator in an infant with long QT syndrome and isolated noncompaction of the ventricular myocardium. Pediatr Cardiol. 2013;34:189–93.
55. Nakashima K, Kusakawa I, Yamamoto T, et al. A left ventricular noncompaction in a patient with long QT syndrome caused by a KCNQ1 mutation: a case report. Heart Vessel. 2013;28:126–9.
56. Nascimento BR, Vidigal DF, Carneiro RD, et al. Complete atrioventricular block as the first manifestation of noncompaction of the ventricular myocardium. Pacing Clin Electrophysiol. 2013;36:e107–10.

57. Ulusoy RE, Kucukarslan N, Kirilmaz A, Demiralp E. Noncompaction of ventricular myocardium involving both ventricles. Eur J Echocardiogr. 2006;7:457–60.
58. Williams T, Machann W, Kuhler L, Hamm H, Müller-Höcker J, Zimmer M, Ertl G, Ritter O, Beer M, Schönberger J. Novel desmoplakin mutation: juvenile biventricular cardiomyopathy with left ventricular non-compaction and acantholytic palmoplantar keratoderma. Clin Res Cardiol. 2011;100:1087–93.
59. Wlodarska EK, Wozniak O, Konka M, Piotrowska-Kownacka D, Walczak E, Hoffman P. Isolated ventricular noncompaction mimicking arrhythmogenic right ventricular cardiomyopathy--a study of nine patients. Int J Cardiol. 2010;145:107–11.
60. Hughes ML, Carstensen B, Wilkinson JL, Weintraub RG. Angiographic diagnosis, prevalence and outcomes for left ventricular noncompaction in children with congenital cardiac disease. Cardiol Young. 2007;17:56–63.
61. Jenni R, Oechslin E, Schneider J, Attenhofer Jost C, Kaufmann PA. Echocardiographic and pathoanatomical characteristics of isolated left ventricular non-compaction: a step towards classification as a distinct cardiomyopathy. Heart. 2001;86:666–71.
62. Oechslin E, Jenni R. Left ventricular non-compaction revisited: a distinct phenotype with genetic heterogeneity? Eur Heart J. 2011;32:1446–56.
63. Punn R, Silverman NH. Cardiac segmental analysis in left ventricular noncompaction: experience in a pediatric population. J Am Soc Echocardiogr. 2010;23:46–53.
64. McMahon CJ, Pignatelli RH, Nagueh SF, et al. Left ventricular non-compaction cardiomyopathy in children: characterisation of clinical status using tissue Doppler-derived indices of left ventricular diastolic relaxation. Heart. 2007;93:676–81.
65. Eidem BW. Noninvasive evaluation of left ventricular noncompaction: what's new in 2009? Pediatr Cardiol. 2009;30:682–9.
66. van Dalen BM, Caliskan K, Soliman OI, et al. Left ventricular solid body rotation in noncompaction cardiomyopathy: a potential new objective and quantitative functional diagnostic criterion? Eur J Heart Fail. 2008;10:1088–93.
67. Petersen SE, Selvanayagam JB, Wiesmann F, et al. Left ventricular non-compaction: insights from cardiovascular magnetic resonance imaging. J Am Coll Cardiol. 2005;46:101–5.
68. Thuny F, Jacquier A, Jop B, et al. Assessment of left ventricular non-compaction in adults: side-by-side comparison of cardiac magnetic resonance imaging with echocardiography. Arch Cardiovasc Dis. 2010;103:150–9.
69. Jacquier A, Thuny F, Jop B, et al. Measurement of trabeculated left ventricular mass using cardiac magnetic resonance imaging in the diagnosis of left ventricular non-compaction. Eur Heart J. 2010;31:1098–104.
70. Uribe S, Cadavid L, Hussain T, et al. Cardiovascular magnetic resonance findings in a pediatric population with isolated left ventricular non-compaction. J Cardiovasc Magn Reson. 2012;14:9.
71. Paterick TE, Tajik AJ. Left ventricular noncompaction a diagnostically challenging cardiomyopathy. Circ J. 2012;76:1556–62.
72. Melendez-Ramirez G, Castillo-Castellon F, Espinola-Zavaleta N, Meave A, Kimura-Hayama ET. Left ventricular noncompaction: a proposal of new diagnostic criteria by multidetector computed tomography. J Cardiovasc Comput Tomogr. 2012;6:346–54.
73. Hollingsworth CL, Yoshizumi TT, Frush DP, et al. Pediatric cardiac-gated CT angiography: assessment of radiation dose. Am J Roentgenol. 2007;189:12–8.
74. Nihei K, Shinomiya N, Kabayama H, et al. Wolff-Parkinson-White (WPW) syndrome in isolated noncompaction of the ventricular myocardium (INVM). Circ J. 2004;68:82–4.
75. Caliskan K, Szili-Torok T, Theuns DA, et al. Indications and outcome of implantable cardioverter-defibrillators for primary and secondary prophylaxis in patients with noncompaction cardiomyopathy. J Cardiovasc Electrophysiol. 2011;22:898–904.
76. Kobza R, Steffel J, Erne P, et al. Implantable cardioverter-defibrillator and cardiac resynchronization therapy in patients with left ventricular noncompaction. Heart Rhythm. 2010;7:1545–9.

77. Van Malderen S, Wijchers S, Akca F, Caliskan K, Szili-Torok T. Mismatch between the origin of premature ventricular complexes and the noncompacted myocardium in patients with noncompaction cardiomyopathy patients: involvement of the conduction system? Ann Noninvasive Electrocardiol. 2016. https://doi.org/10.1111/anec.12394. [Epub ahead of print].
78. Jefferies JL, Wilkinson JD, Sleeper LA, et al. Cardiomyopathy phenotypes and outcomes for children with left ventricular myocardial noncompaction: Results from the Pediatric Cardiomyopathy Registry. J Card Fail. 2015;21(11):877–84.
79. van Waning JI, Caliskan K, Hoedemaekers YM, et al. Genetics, clinical features, and long-term outcome of noncompaction cardiomyopathy. J Am Coll Cardiol. 2018;71(7):711–22.
80. Sasse-Klaassen S, Gerull B, Oechslin E, Jenni R, Thierfelder L. Isolated noncompaction of the left ventricular myocardium in the adult is an autosomal dominant disorder in the majority of patients. Am J Med Genet A. 2003;119A:162–7.
81. Digilio M, Bernardini L, Gagliardi M, et al. Syndromic non-compaction of the left ventricle: associated chromosomal anomalies. Clin Genet. 2013;84(4):362–7.
82. Beken S, Cevik A, Turan O, et al. A neonatal case of left ventricular noncompaction associated with trisomy 18. Genet Couns. 2011;22(2):161–4.
83. Yukifumi M, Hirohiko S, Fukiko I, Mariko M. Trisomy 13 in a 9-year-old girl with left ventricular noncompaction. Pediatr Cardiol. 2011;32(2):206–7.
84. Blinder JJ, Martinez HR, Craigen WJ, Belmont J, Pignatelli RH, Jefferies JL. Noncompaction of the left ventricular myocardium in a boy with a novel chromosome 8p23.1 deletion. Am J Med Genet A. 2011;155A(9):2215–20.
85. Martinez HR, Niu MC, Sutton VR, et al. Coffin-Lowry syndrome and left ventricular noncompaction cardiomyopathy with a restrictive pattern. Am J Med Genet A. 2011;155A(12):3030–4.
86. Martinez HR, Belmont JW, Craigen WJ, Taylor MD, Jefferies JL. Left ventricular noncompaction in Sotos syndrome. Am J Med Genet A. 2011;155A(5):1115–8.
87. Zechner U, Kohlschmidt N, Kempf O, et al. Familial Sotos syndrome caused by a novel missense mutation, C2175S, in NSD1 and associated with normal intelligence, insulin dependent diabetes, bronchial asthma, and lipedema. Eur J Med Genet. 2009;52(5):306–10.
88. Sellars EA, Zimmerman SL, Smolarek T, Hopkin RJ. Ventricular noncompaction and absent thumbs in a newborn with tetrasomy 5q35.2-5q35.3: an association with Hunter-McAlpine syndrome? Am J Med Genet A. 2011;155A(6):1409–13.
89. Corrado G, Checcarelli N, Santarone M, Stollberger C, Finsterer J. Left ventricular hypertrabeculation/noncompaction with PMP22 duplication-based Charcot-Marie-Tooth disease type 1A. Cardiology. 2006;105(3):142–5.
90. Klaassen S, Probst S, Oechslin E, et al. Mutations in sarcomere protein genes in left ventricular noncompaction. Circulation. 2008;117:2893–901.
91. Hoedemaekers YM, Caliskan K, Michels M, et al. The importance of genetic counseling, DNA diagnostics, and cardiologic family screening in left ventricular noncompaction cardiomyopathy. Circ Cardiovasc Genet. 2010;3:232–9.
92. Miller EM, Hinton RB, Czosek R, Lorts A, Parrott A, Shikany AR, Ittenbach RF, Ware SM. Genetic testing in pediatric left ventricular noncompaction. Circ Cardiovasc Genet. 2017;10(6). pii: e001735. https://doi.org/10.1161/CIRCGENETICS.117.001735.
93. Towbin JA, Jefferies JL. Cardiomyopathies Due to Left Ventricular Noncompaction, Mitochondrial and Storage Diseases, and Inborn Errors of Metabolism. Circ Res. 2017;21:838–54.
94. Finsterer J, Stöllberger C, Towbin JA. Left ventricular noncompaction cardiomyopathy: cardiac, neuromuscular, and genetic factors. Nat Rev Cardiol. 2017;14:224–37.
95. Parent JJ, Towbin JA, Jefferies JL. Left ventricular noncompaction in a family with lamin A/C gene mutation. Tex Heart Inst J. 2015;42:73–6.
96. Shan L, Makita N, Xing Y, et al. SCN5A variants in Japanese patients with left ventricular noncompaction and arrhythmia. Mol Genet Metab. 2008;93:468–74.
97. Towbin JA. Ion channel dysfunction associated with arrhythmia, ventricular noncompaction, and mitral valve prolapse a new overlapping phenotype. J Am Coll Cardiol. 2014;64(8):768–71.

98. Schweizer PA, Schröter J, Greiner S, Haas J, Yampolsky P, Mereles D, Buss SJ, Seyler C, Bruehl C, Draguhn A, Koenen M, Meder B, Katus HA, Thomas D. The symptom complex of familial sinus node dysfunction and myocardial noncompaction is associated with mutations in the HCN4 channel. J Am Coll Cardiol. 2014;64(8):757–67.
99. Milano A, Vermeer AM, Lodder EM, Barc J, Verkerk AO, Postma AV, van der Bilt IA, Baars MJ, van Haelst PL, Caliskan K, Hoedemaekers YM, Le Scouarnec S, Redon R, Pinto YM, Christiaans I, Wilde AA, Bezzina CR. HCN4 mutations in multiple families with bradycardia and left ventricular noncompaction cardiomyopathy. J Am Coll Cardiol. 2014;64(8):745–56.
100. Towbin JA, Lorts A, Jefferies JL. Left ventricular non-compaction cardiomyopathy. Lancet. 2015;386(9995):813–25.
101. Bleyl SB, Mumford BR, Brown-Harrison MC, et al. Xq28-linked noncompaction of the left ventricular myocardium: prenatal diagnosis and pathologic analysis of affected individuals. Am J Med Genet. 1997;72(3):257–65.
102. Ouyang P, Saarel E, Bai Y, et al. A de novo mutation in NKX2.5 associated with atrial septal defects, ventricular noncompaction, syncope and sudden death. Clin Chim Acta. 2011;412:170–5.
103. Postma AV, van Engelen K, van de Meerakker J, et al. Mutations in the sarcomere gene MYH7 in Ebstein anomaly. Circ Cardiovasc Genet. 2011;4:43–50.
104. Kelle AM, Bentley SJ, Rohena LO, Cabalka AK, Olson TM. Ebstein anomaly, left ventricular non-compaction, and early onset heart failure associated with a de novo α-tropomyosin gene mutation. Am J Med Genet A. 2016;170(8):2186–90.
105. Probst S, Oechslin E, Schuler P, et al. Sarcomere gene mutations in isolated left ventricular noncompaction cardiomyopathy do not predict clinical phenotype. Circ Cardiovasc Genet. 2011;4:367–74.
106. Dellefave LM, Pytel P, Mewborn S, et al. Sarcomere mutations in cardiomyopathy with left ventricular hypertrabeculation. Circ Cardiovasc Genet. 2009;2:442–9.
107. Hastings R, de Villiers CP, Hooper C, et al. Combination of whole genome sequencing, linkage, and functional studies implicates a missense mutation in titin as a cause of autosomal dominant cardiomyopathy with features of left ventricular noncompaction. Circ Cardiovasc Genet. 2016;9:426–35.
108. Bagnall RD, Molloy LK, Kalman JM, Semsarian C. Exome sequencing identifies a mutation in the ACTN2 gene in a family with idiopathic ventricular fibrillation, left ventricular non-compaction, and sudden death. BMC Med Genet. 2014;15:99.
109. Finsterer J, Stollberger C. Primary myopathies and the heart. Scand Cardiovasc J. 2008;42:9–24.
110. Ramond F, Janin A, Di Filippo S, et al. Homozygous PKP2 deletion associated with neonatal left ventricle noncompaction. Clin Genet. 2017;91:126–30.
111. Tang S, Batra A, Zhang Y, Ebenroth ES, Huang T. Left ventricular noncompaction is associated with mutations in the mitochondrial genome. Mitochondrion. 2010;10:350–7.
112. Arndt AK, Schafer S, Drenckhahn JD, et al. Fine mapping of the 1p36 deletion syndrome identifies mutation of PRDM16 as a cause of cardiomyopathy. Am J Hum Genet. 2013;93:67–77.
113. Pearce FB, Litovsky SH, Dabal RJ, et al. Pathologic features of dilated cardiomyopathy with localized noncompaction in a child with deletion 1p36 syndrome. Congenit Heart Dis. 2012;7:59–61.
114. Teekakirikul P, Kelly MA, Rehm HL, Lakdawala NK, Funke BH. Inherited cardiomyopathies: molecular genetics and clinical genetic testing in the postgenomic era. J Mol Diagn. 2013;15:158–70.
115. Schreiber SL, Crabtree GR. Immunophilins, ligands, and the control of signal transduction. Harvey Lect. 1995;91:99–114.
116. Wang T, Donahoe PK. The immunophilin FKBP12: a molecular guardian of the TGF-beta family type I receptors. Front Biosci. 2004;9:619–31.

117. Cameron AM, Steiner JP, Roskams AJ, Ali SM, Ronnett GV, Snyder SH. Calcineurin associated with the inositol 1,4,5-trisphosphate receptor-FKBP12 complex modulates Ca2+ flux. Cell. 1995;83:463–72.
118. Maruyama M, Li BY, Chen H, et al. FKBP12 is a critical regulator of the heart rhythm and the cardiac voltage-gated sodium current in mice. Circ Res. 2011;108:1042–52.
119. Shou W, Aghdasi B, Armstrong DL, et al. Cardiac defects and altered ryanodine receptor function in mice lacking FKBP12. Nature. 1998;391:489–92.
120. Chen H, Zhang W, Sun X, et al. Fkbp1a controls ventricular myocardium trabeculation and compaction by regulating endocardial Notch1 activity. Development. 2013;140:1946–57.
121. Luxan G, Casanova JC, Martinez-Poveda B, et al. Mutations in the NOTCH pathway regulator MIB1 cause left ventricular noncompaction cardiomyopathy. Nat Med. 2013;19:193–201.
122. Chen H, Shi S, Acosta L, et al. BMP10 is essential for maintaining cardiac growth during murine cardiogenesis. Development. 2004;131:2219–31.
123. Zhao C, Guo H, Li J, et al. Numb family proteins are essential for cardiac morphogenesis and progenitor differentiation. Development. 2014;141:281–95.
124. Pashmforoush M, Lu JT, Chen H, et al. Nkx2-5 pathways and congenital heart disease; loss of ventricular myocyte lineage specification leads to progressive cardiomyopathy and complete heart block. Cell. 2004;117:373–86.
125. Ashraf H, Pradhan L, Chang EI, et al. A mouse model of human congenital heart disease: high incidence of diverse cardiac anomalies and ventricular noncompaction produced by heterozygous Nkx2-5 homeodomain missense mutation. Circ Cardiovasc Genet. 2014;7:423–33.
126. Chen Q, Chen H, Zheng D, et al. Smad7 is required for the development and function of the heart. J Biol Chem. 2009;284:292–300.
127. Liu J, Farmer JD Jr, Lane WS, Friedman J, Weissman I, Schreiber SL. Calcineurin is a common target of cyclophilin-cyclosporin A and FKBP-FK506 complexes. Cell. 1991;66:807–15.
128. de la Pompa JL, Timmerman LA, Takimoto H, et al. Role of the NF-ATc transcription factor in morphogenesis of cardiac valves and septum. Nature. 1998;392:182–6.
129. Whetstine JR, Nottke A, Lan F, et al. Reversal of histone lysine trimethylation by the JMJD2 family of histone demethylases. Cell. 2006;125:467–81.
130. Shen X, Kim W, Fujiwara Y, et al. Jumonji modulates polycomb activity and self-renewal versus differentiation of stem cells. Cell. 2009;139:1303–14.
131. Landeira D, Sauer S, Poot R, et al. Jarid2 is a PRC2 component in embryonic stem cells required for multi-lineage differentiation and recruitment of PRC1 and RNA Polymerase II to developmental regulators. Nat Cell Biol. 2010;12:618–24.
132. Mysliwiec MR, Bresnick EH, Lee Y. Endothelial Jarid2/Jumonji is required for normal cardiac development and proper Notch1 expression. J Biol Chem. 2011;286:17193–204.
133. Grego-Bessa J, Luna-Zurita L, del Monte G, et al. Notch signaling is essential for ventricular chamber development. Dev Cell. 2007;12:415–29.
134. Jefferies JL. Barth syndrome. Am J Med Genet C Semin Med Genet. 2013;163:198–205.
135. Phoon CK, Acehan D, Schlame M, et al. Tafazzin knockdown in mice leads to a developmental cardiomyopathy with early diastolic dysfunction preceding myocardial noncompaction. J Am Heart Assoc. 2012;1. pii: jah3-e000455. https://doi.org/10.1161/JAHA.111.000455.
136. Yancy CW, Jessup M, Bozkurt B, et al. 2013 ACCF/AHA guideline for the management of heart failure: a report of the American College of Cardiology Foundation/American Heart Association Task Force on Practice Guidelines. J Am Coll Cardiol. 2013;62:e147–239.
137. Gersh BJ, Maron BJ, Bonow RO, et al. American College of Cardiology Foundation/American Heart Association Task Force on Practice Guidelines. 2011 ACCF/AHA Guideline for the Diagnosis and Treatment of Hypertrophic Cardiomyopathy: a report of the American College of Cardiology Foundation/American Heart Association Task Force on Practice Guidelines. Developed in collaboration with the American Association for Thoracic Surgery, American Society of Echocardiography, American Society of Nuclear Cardiology, Heart Failure Society of America, Heart Rhythm Society, Society for Cardiovascular Angiography and Interventions, and Society of Thoracic Surgeons. J Am Coll Cardiol. 2011;58:e212–60.
138. Pitta S, Thatai D, Afonso L. Thromboembolic complications of left ventricular noncompaction: case report and brief review of the literature. J Clin Ultrasound. 2007;35:465–8.

Genetics and Family Screening for Noncompaction Cardiomyopathy

8

Jaap I. van Waning and Danielle Majoor-Krakauer

Introduction

Noncompaction cardiomyopathy (NCCM) is characterized by endocardial hyper-trabeculation of the myocardium of the left ventricle. In 1997 the first genetic cause for NCCM, a mutation in the X-linked *TAZ* gene, was identified in a family were six boys had Barth syndrome with hypertrabeculation of the left ventricle [1]. The link of familial NCCM to defects in the sarcomere genes that had previously been linked to the more frequent hereditary hypertrophic (HCM) and dilated cardiomyopathies (DCM), came in 2007 by the report of *MYH7* mutations in NCCM and was followed by reports of other sarcomere gene mutations in familial NCCM [2, 3].

In NCCM the sarcomere genes are the most prevalent genetic causes. More recently the introduction of next generation sequencing (NGS), allowing simultaneous analysis of panels of 50 or more cardiomyopathy genes, showed that around 35% of NCCM patients have a mutation, and that mutations occur more frequently in children diagnosed with NCCM than in patients diagnosed as adults [4, 5].

Overall, approximately 50% of NCCM patients are considered to have a genetic cause [4]. Some because they have inherited a mutation in a cardiomyopathy gene, other patients have family members with a cardiomyopathy without having a mutation in a known cardiomyopathy gene. In 45% of familial NCCM no mutation can be identified [4], indicating that many genetic causes for NCCM are still unknown. Overall around 50% of cases diagnosed today with NCCM have no mutation in a cardiomyopathy gene or familial disease. In these -mostly adult patients- NCCM may be attributed to non-genetic, secondary causes for hypertrabeculation. Alternatively, these cases may have yet unknown (complex) genetic cause(s) carrying small risk for relatives [4]. For NCCM, like for HCM and DCM, it is important

J. I. van Waning (✉) · D. Majoor-Krakauer
Department of Clinical Genetics, Erasmus MC University Medical Center,
Rotterdam, The Netherlands
e-mail: j.vanwaning@erasmusmc.nl

© Springer Nature Switzerland AG 2019
K. Caliskan et al. (eds.), *Noncompaction Cardiomyopathy*,
https://doi.org/10.1007/978-3-030-17720-1_8

for relatives of patients to be informed about the increased risk of having a cardiomyopathy.

For that reason referral of patients diagnosed with NCCM for genetic counseling, has become common practice [6]. This allows, by taking family histories and performing DNA testing of the index case, to estimate the risk for relatives to have NCCM. When there is a mutation, DNA testing for the familial mutation of first degree relatives is advised, with subsequent cardiologic screening of mutation carriers. In NCCM genetic defects may predict risk of having severe cardiac events (MACE). Some genes, like *MYH7,* carry lower risk for MACE than other genes. In this perspective DNA testing may help stratify risk for MACE of patient and relatives and help guide clinical management of genetic NCCM accordingly [4]. For families of patients without a mutation, cardiologic screening of first degree relatives is recommended, also in absence of a family history of cardiomyopathy, because we cannot exclude that these patients may have an unknown genetic predisposition with low penetrance that conveys a small risk to relatives.

The aim of this chapter is to give an overview of the genetic causes for NCCM, and describe the routine of genetic diagnostics i.e. genetic counseling, DNA testing and initiating family screening. Illustrating in this way the importance of integrating genetic diagnostics to clinical management of NCCM patients by conveying appropriate information to patients and their families, in order to make early diagnosis and timely treatment accessible for the families of all NCCM patients.

The Genetics of NCCM

Genetics plays a more important role in some patients with hypertrabeculation of the left ventricle than in others. Currently three main categories of genetic burden for noncompaction are recognized (Fig. 8.1). (1) Patients with a genetic

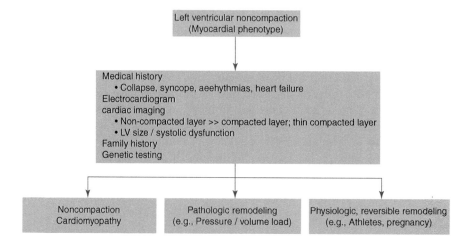

Fig. 8.1 NCCM groups

noncompaction cardiomyopathy. These are the patients with a mutation in a cardiomyopathy gene and/or relatives with a cardiomyopathy (familial cardiomyopathy). In genetic NCCM relatives have an increased risk of having a cardiomyopathy. In 45% of familial NCCM no mutation is found, indicating that not all NCCM genes have been identified yet [4]. The majority of the genes associated with NCCM also play an important role in genetic hypertrophic (HCM) and dilated cardiomyopathy (DCM) [7, 8]. For now, there is no explanation how overlapping genetic defects in these sarcomere genes cause the spectrum of phenotypes ranging from hypertrophic, dilated and noncompaction cardiomyopathy. (2) Cardiomyopathy patients with noncompaction without a genetic cause; in these 'sporadic' NCCM cases no evidence for a genetic cause is found by DNA analysis, and the family history and/or family screening are uninformative. These patients have similar cardiac outcomes as genetic NCCM patients. In sporadic patients NCCM may be the result of pathologic cardiac remodeling, activated by other (now unknown genetic or non-genetic) causes leading to hypertrabeculation. In these patients high incidences of left bundle branch blocks were identified [4]. Also cardiac comorbidities like hypertension may play a role in these patients [4]. We cannot exclude that apparently sporadic patient may have defect in a yet unknown cardiomyopathy gene, since not all cardiomyopathy genes have been identified yet. We know that at least one third of the NCCM patients with a mutation in a cardiomyopathy gene, did not report familial disease, indicating that negative family history does not exclude a genetic cause [4]. Another possibility is that a group of apparently sporadic NCCM patients may have variants in known or unknown cardiomyopathy genes that have insufficient genetic effects and need additional interaction with other genetic or non-genetic factors to cause NCCM. (3) Healthy individuals with a benign LV hypertrabeculation; large population based studies have reported that LV hypertrabeculation may occur as frequently as in 43% of the healthy adult population [9]. A higher susceptibility for having more prominent trabeculations, without features of a cardiomyopathy was reported in blacks and athletes [10, 11]. The cause might be a genetic or epigenetic regulation of gene expression or translation, activating similar pathways as mutations in sarcomere genes, causing hypertrabeculation without cardiomyopathy. The high incidence of hypertrabeculation supports that the currently used echo and MRI diagnostic criteria, relying on the ratio between noncompacted and compacted layer of myocardium, cannot distinguish pathologic noncompaction cardiomyopathy from benign, sometimes reversible, left ventricle hypertrabeculation without cardiomyopathy and therefore more sensitive diagnostic criteria are needed.

NCCM Genes

In familial NCCM around 55% of NCCM patients have a mutation, indicating that the genetic cause has not been found for a large proportion of familial NCCM [4]. In children and in adult patients the majority of the mutations occur in genes encoding for proteins of the cardiac sarcomere structure and function (Fig. 8.2) [4]. Less frequent genetic causes for NCCM are defects in genes encoding for intracellular signaling, homeostasis and cytoskeletal integrity associated with NCCM [12]. Genetic causes are identified more frequently in patients diagnosed in childhood than in adults with NCCM [4]. These observations show how little we understand about the development of the hypertrabeculation, because they suggest that the genetic effects might involve cardiac development as well as cardiac remodeling at older age.

Genes for Autosomal Dominant Inherited NCCM

Defects in sarcomere genes are the most common genetic cause for NCCM (Fig. 8.2) [4]. These forms of NCCM have an autosomal dominant inheritance pattern. Patients (usually) inherited the mutation from one of the parents. Siblings and offspring of these patients have a 50% risk of having inherited the familial mutation. Reduced penetrance is a well-known feature of sarcomere mutations in genetic cardiomyopathies [13], meaning that for unknown reasons, around 30% (the percentage may vary by gene and variant) of the carriers (i.e. relatives with the familial mutation) do not have a cardiomyopathy. In a small proportion (4%) of the patients the mutation has occurred de novo [4, 14]. In that case the mutation is not inherited from the parents and there is no increased risk for siblings, although risk for offspring of having the mutations remains 50%. Compound heterozygosity for sarcomere mutations, occurs when a patient inherited a (different) mutation from each parent. This is not very rare, since sarcomere mutations occur relatively frequently in the population [15]. Patients with two sarcomere gene mutations may have more severe clinical features than their relatives with single mutations [16]. In NCCM the most frequent genetic causes (71%) are defects in sarcomere genes: *MYH7*, *TTN* and *MYBPC3*. Less frequently (11%) affected are the other sarcomere genes: *ACTC1*, *LDB3*, *TNNC1*, *TNNI3* and *TNNT2*. Rare genetic causes are the other autosomal dominantly inherited cardiomyopathy genes *CASQ2*, *HCN4*, *KCNH2*, *KCNQ1*,

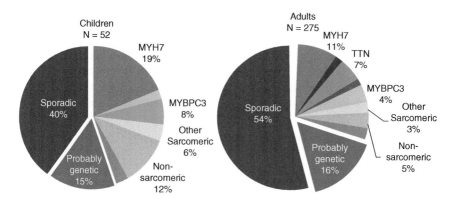

Darker shades indicate complex genotypes. DNA testing of approximately 45 cardiomyopathy genes and family histories showed that children were more likely to have a mutation.

Fig. 8.2 Mutation frequencies

RYR2 and *SCN5A,* involved in ion transport and genes affecting other cardiomyocyte functions or structure like, *CSRP3, DSP, LMNA, MIB1, MIB2* and *PLN* [4, 5], occurring altogether in approximately 6% of the patients.

Genes for X-linked Inherited NCCM

Defects of genes on the X chromosome affect only males and are inherited in an X linked pattern. With this type of inheritance sons of unaffected female carriers have 50% risk of being affected. Daughters of patients or of female carriers have 50% risk of being an (unaffected) carrier and transmitting the trait to their sons. Barth syndrome is caused by defects in the *TAZ* gene on the X chromosome. Among the other X-linked causes for NCCM are some genes causing neuromuscular disorders, *DMD, EMD, FHL1, GLA, LAMP2,*and rare neurodevelopmental disorders caused by mutations in the *NONO,* and *RPS6KA3* genes [17].

Genes for Autosomal Recessive Inherited NCCM

Recessive inherited NCCM is rare and was reported in single childhood cases with inborn errors of metabolism, related to a *FKTN* or *SDHD* mutation [18, 19].

Mitochondrial Defects and NCCM

Mitochondrial disorders are caused by defects in the mitochondrial (Mt) DNA or by a defect in nuclear DNA genes encoding for structures of the mitochondria. Defects in Mt genes are passed on cytoplasmatically in germ cells from mother to child. Defects in nuclear genes have dominant, recessive or X-linked inheritance pattern. Mutations in genes affecting the mitochondrial functioning lead to insufficient energy production required in various organs, particularly those with high energy demands, like the central nervous system, skeletal and cardiac muscles. These disorders present with a wide spectrum of clinical features including cardiomyopathy, visual impairment, deafness, stroke, epilepsy and diabetes. Mt. genes linked to NCCM are *MT-ATP6, MT-ATP8, MT-CO1, MT-CO3, MT-CYB, MT-ND1, MT-ND2* and *MT-ND6* [20, 21]. Nuclear genes coding for the mitochondria linked to NCCM are *DNAJC19, GARS, HADHB, MIPEP, MTFMT* and *NNT* [22]. To find Mt gene defects a specific analysis of the Mt DNA and nuclear DNA is needed, since these genes are not routinely sequenced in NGS cardiomyopathy gene panels.

Chromosomal Defects

A number of chromosomal deletions and duplications have been associated with NCCM. These chromosomal defects are usually identified in children. Because they affect multiple genes they lead to complex congenital malformation syndromes. The 1p36 deletion syndrome is frequently reported presenting with NCCM, intellectual disability, delayed growth, hypotonia, seizures, limited speech ability, hearing and vision impairment and distinct facial features [23]. Other chromosome anomalies linked to NCCM are deletions of 1q, 5q35, 7p21, 8p23.1, 22q11 and Xq28 [24]. In addition NCCM has been observed in monosomy X (Turner syndrome) and trisomy 13, trisomy 18, trisomy 21 and trisomy 22 patients [25]. To detect a small chromosome anomaly, an array analysis has to be performed, since these defects are not recognized by NGS sequencing of cardiomyopathy genes.

Genetic Counseling and Genetic Diagnosis of NCCM

Genetic counseling is recommended for all patients fulfilling diagnostic criteria for NCCM to perform DNA analysis and detect familial disease. This information is needed to estimate risk for relatives, convey information on the risks to index cases and their families and subsequently initiate family screening. Like in HCM and DCM family screening for NCCM is recommended because it allows accurate and timely diagnosis of NCCM improving prognosis of patients in the family. To initiate genetic diagnostics for NCCM, index patients are counseled about the consequences of the results of DNA testing, and an informed consent for DNA testing is requested.

Genetic counseling involves communicating the goal of genetic testing and the explaining the importance of informing family members. Genetic counselors are trained to explain the clinical features of the disease and the inheritance pattern, to the index case and organize informing and screening family members. Genetic counseling has grown out of the need to personalize scientific information and to translate it into a user-friendly language that is accessible intellectually and emotionally for the patient and its family. Helping index cases and their relatives—if necessary-to handle the information on heredity, and discuss the subsequent risks and consequences, is an important part of the process of genetic counseling. The routine for genetic diagnosis and family screening for NCCM is summarized in Fig. 8.3. It is hereby the role of the genetic counselor to identify and help, during pre- and post-test counseling, coping with adverse feelings that some patients or relatives may experience like distress, anxiety or guilt, evoked by the possibility of a genetic cause for NCCM [26]. It is important, in particular for asymptomatic relatives, to discuss that having a genetic risk and having a choice of predictive testing, whether by DNA analysis or cardiologic exam, may have medical implications, as well as psychological and socio -economic consequences. The genetic counselor may offer access to specialized psychologic support when needed by families.

Family History

At the departments of clinical genetics information on the occurrence of cardiomyopathies in the family of NCCM patients is obtained, and medical records of affected relatives are retrieved for verification of the diagnosis, when possible. Family

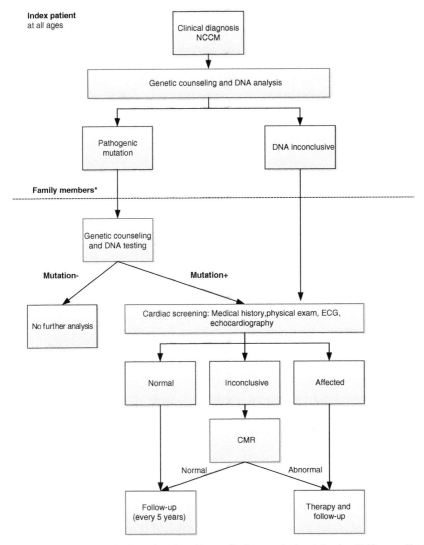

*Presymptomatic DNA testing for relatives above 18 years. Cardiac screening for relatives from10-12 years, without DNA testing. DNA testing if cardiomyopathies is identified at all ages.
In blue: at the clinical genetics departement
In red: at the cardiology departement

Fig. 8.3 Flowchart screening

history taking helps to determine if cardiomyopathy is familial and to identify the mode of inheritance [27]. It is importance to acknowledge that an uninformative family history cannot completely exclude a genetic cause for NCCM. Because around 20% of NCCM patients without affected relatives had a mutation [4]. The reasons for underreporting of familial cardiomyopathy might be that affected relatives might not have been diagnosed with NCCM. It is known that approximately 30% of the NCCM patients have a cardiomyopathy without the typical symptoms of cardiomyopathy at time of diagnosis [28]. Also, like in HCM, non-penetrance occurs in around 30% of the carriers of a familial (sarcomere) mutations and these carriers do not have a cardiomyopathy [28]. Another explanation for underreporting familial disease may be that family histories are not informative when families are small or patients have little information on relatives. Important questions when taking a family history for the purpose of establishing whether there is a familial cardiomyopathy is asking if relatives have had heart failure, arrhythmias, accidental or unexpected deaths, thromboses (including stroke), any kind of cardiac surgery, or if they had a congenital heart defect or neuromuscular disease. When family screening is performed the family histories are adjusted according to the results of the DNA and cardiac screening of relatives.

DNA Testing for NCCM

The purpose of DNA testing—irrespective of the age of the patient—is to identify the genetic cause for NCCM [4, 5]. An important aspect of DNA testing is that finding a mutation allows asymptomatic relatives to have a predictive DNA test that identifies accurately which relatives have a mutation and have an increased risk of developing a cardiomyopathy. In this way identifying the causative mutation facilitates genetic cascade screening. In families with a mutation, relatives who do not carry the familial mutation can be excluded from regular cardiac follow-up and can be reassured that there is no increased risk for their offspring. DNA testing may help to confirm the diagnosis for patient with borderline features of NCCM. In addition as we have shown recently, the genotype (specific genetic defect) may help to predict risk for ventricular systolic dysfunction and major cardiac adverse events for patients and guide clinical management accordingly [4], as discussed in more detail in the paragraph on *genotype-phenotype correlations*.

NGS Cardiomyopathy Gene Panels

Since a large number of genes are involved in NCCM, the application of novel methods of DNA analysis like NGS and exome based testing has been proven to improve the yield of genetic testing with the simultaneous analysis of panels with large numbers of cardiomyopathy genes [3]. Current cardiomyopathy gene panels used in diagnostic and commercial laboratories may include the following genes: *ABCC9, **ACTC1, ACTN2**, ANKRD1, BAG3, CALR3, CRYAB, CSRP3, DES, **DMD**, DSC2, DSG2, **DSP, EMD, GLA**, JPH2, JUP, LAMA4, **LAMP2, LDB3, LMNA, MYBPC3**, MYH6, **MYH7**, MYL2, MYL3, **MYPN**, MYOZ1, MYOZ2, **PKP2, PLN**, PRKAG2, **RBM20**, RYR2, SCN5A, SGCD, TAZ, TCAP, TMEM43, **TNNC1, TNNI3, TNNT2, TPM1, TTN** and VCL* (in bold the genes that were associated so far with NCCM). These genes encode proteins constituting structure and function of the sarcomere, cytoskeleton, desmosome, ion channels or nuclear lamina, and proteins participating in Ca2+ handling during contraction phase of action potential of the cardiomyocyte or affecting cardiac energy metabolism and are related to a large spectrum of cardiomyopathies. In case a cardiomyopathy gene panel is not available, DNA testing for NCCM of a smaller number of genes including *MYH7*, *MYBPC3* and *TTN,* which have a large proportion of the genetic defects in NCCM, is advised.

Gene Variant Classification System

For a correct interpretation of the results of DNA analysis stringent novel guidelines for classification of genetic variants are applied since 2015 [29]. The outcome of DNA analysis for clinical purpose are currently classified into pathogenic variants (PV), likely pathogenic variants (LPV), variants of unknown clinical significance (VUS), likely benign or benign variants. This classification system for variants is based on in silico prediction of pathogenicity, population frequencies and previous reports providing (functional) evidence of the pathogenic nature of the specific variants [30]. Variants classified as PV or LPV in sarcomere genes are usually nonsynonymous substitutions or deletions of a nucleotide classified as missense, nonsense, or frameshift mutations and have a deleterious effect on the protein. Older results of DNA testing should be re-evaluated, because some of the variants previously reported as (pathogenic) mutations may now be reclassified as not pathogenic. Application of novel classification system to a large number of variants in sarcomere genes in NCCM patients showed recently that 50% of variants previously reported to be pathogenic, were reclassified as VUS or benign variants [31]. Similarly a large proportion of variants reported previously as mutations in sarcomere genes in HCM patients, were reclassified recently as VUS or benign variants [32]. This endorses that the continuous surveillance of variant classification is needed, because new evidence on DNA variants like population frequencies, results of novel functional tests or in silico predictor tools comes out [33]. DNA testing of pre-symptomatic family members is only indicated when there is a PV or LPV in the family. Since the effect of VUS is not known, these variants cannot reliably predict risk for NCCM in relatives and therefor these variants are not of used for family screening.

DNA Testing of NCCM Patients with CHD, Neuromuscular Disease or NCCM with Multiple Congenital Anomalies Syndrome

Around 10% of NCCM patients have a concomitant congenital heart defect [34]. Some families with NCCM and Ebstein anomaly, have a mutation in *MYH7* [35]. There is little evidence that the combination of NCCM with other forms of CHD segregate in families or are caused by specific genetic defects. Thus it remains unknown if there are common (epi)genetic causes affecting embryologic cardiac development explaining the co-occurrence of NCCM and CHD, or that they co-occur by coincidence. NCCM in some patients represent cardiac manifestations of inherited neuromuscular disorders, for which specific diagnostic gene panels need to be requested since these genes are usually not included in the regular cardiomyopathy gene panels [36]. Also NCCM patients with multiple congenital malformations, usually children, need additional DNA testing and/ or chromosome analysis (array). According to clinical features, that may include screening for mitochondrial defects or metabolic disorders occurring predominantly in childhood NCCM.

Family Screening

Risk for Cardiomyopathy in Relatives

Overall affected relatives of NCCM patients have less severe cardiac features than the index cases, and relatives of index cases with a mutation have more risk of having a cardiomyopathy than the relatives of cases without a mutation. Because, at diagnosis affected relatives have usually less attenuated cardiac symptoms than the index case, independent of age at diagnosis, since most relatives are asymptomatic [28]. And some of the index cases without a mutation may have a non-genetic, secondary cause for NCCM, with lower risk for relatives. The risk for relatives of having a cardiomyopathy is furthermore related to the genetic defect in the index case, the mode of inheritance, the gene specific penetrance and—chance of having asymptomatic disease. These factors and also the age at diagnosis of the index case may help to determine the genetic risk for relatives. Also family history of cardiomyopathy or sudden cardiac death in the family may add information about the genetic risk for relatives. It is important for relatives to know that carriers of a familial mutation may have no signs of cardiomyopathy at cardiologic examination. Non-penetrance was observed in 17% of carriers of familial *MHY7* mutations, 33% of carriers of *MYBPC3* and 28% of carriers of *TTN* mutations [28]. Intrafamilial variability of cardiac features is a well-known feature of familial cardiomyopathies. The left ventricle (LV) dimension of the NCCM index case may be a predictor for disease severity in relatives. The dimension of the LV in NCCM relatives corresponded significantly with the LV phenotype of the index case. In addition, since the LV dimension in NCCM patients was related to the course of the disease, the LV function may predict severity for relatives. Patients with NCCM and normal LV-dimensions had a mild course of the disease, with less frequent LV-systolic dysfunction or cardiac events. Patients with NCCM with a dilated LV-dimensions (like in DCM), had a more severe disease course with frequent LV-systolic dysfunction and adverse events. In the families of NCCM patients, 20% of the affected relatives have HCM or DCM without signs of hypertrabeculation [28]. In addition relatives of NCCM patients may have an increased risk for CHD, compared to population risk [28].

Screening Adult Relatives of NCCM Patients

In families with a causative mutation, adult relatives can be offered predictive DNA testing. Predictive DNA testing of relatives can reliably identify which relatives carry a mutation and have an increased risk of developing a cardiomyopathy and thus need clinical surveillance. Relatives who do not carry the mutation can be excluded from regular cardiac follow-up and also can be reassured that there is no increased risk for cardiomyopathy for their offspring.

In families without a mutation, cardiologic family screening of first-degree relatives is recommended. Family screening can be initiated by asking the index patients to distribute a letter to their first and second-degree relatives with information on counseling for genetic risk for NCCM and recommendations for predictive DNA and/or cardiologic family screening. The legal framework for informing relatives varies, in most countries it is the index patient and not the clinician, who must inform relatives and invite them for screening on behalf of the healthcare system [37]. It is important that relatives consent and are correctly informed, *before* they are tested, about the risk of having a cardiomyopathy and about the eventual consequences when they are carriers of a familial mutation and/or signs of cardiomyopathy are detected at cardiologic exam. Diagnosis of a mutation or a cardiomyopathy, even when a relative is asymptomatic may have medical, psychologically as well as socio- economically consequences. For instance regarding life insurance, pension, life style (sporting activities), and eligibility for fostering and adoption [38]. Most relatives have no symptoms of cardiomyopathy and have not been diagnosed when they have a predictive DNA test or have the first cardiologic examination. One of the reasons relatives may choose to have a predictive test is that they want to be in control of their life and gain clarity. Others, doubt wanting to have disclosure, because they believe they may be better of not knowing about the risk giving the chance of being asymptomatic for years. A genetic counselor can help to guide in their decisions to have a pre-symptomatic test.

Screening Young Relatives for NCCM

Like in other age dependent hereditary cardiomyopathies, the recommendations for pre-symptomatic screening are not the same for adults and children. Cardiologic screening is usually recommended from the age that first symptoms may appear. For instance for HCM, cardiologic screening starts around 10–12 years for asymptomatic children with unknown genetic status [38]. In practice these guidelines are followed for NCCM as well. In families with a mutation, predictive DNA testing in children is usually postponed until the age that they can make an informed decision. Because the medical benefit of pre-symptomatic DNA diagnosis of having a familial mutation has not been established for children. The main advantage of pre-symptomatic DNA testing of children is that when a familial mutation can be excluded the child can be discharged from life-long follow-up. In contrast, for the asymptomatic children who are found to be carriers of a familial mutation, recommendations include regular cardiologic follow-up and address life style, like refraining from competitive sports [38]. The burden for children of regular hospital visits, may have adverse psychological like anxiety or depression and may harm a child's self-esteem [39, 40]. Another adverse effect of pre-symptomatic testing in children and adults alike are possible economic disadvantages like higher life insurance or mortgages later in life. For that reason predictive DNA testing for a familial mutation is usually performed in relatives above the age of 18 years. Clinical and/or genetic screening should be considered from younger age if the child has symptoms which can point to a cardiomyopathy or in families with a history of early-onset cardiomyopathy.

Pregnancy and Prenatal Testing

An important aspect of the counseling and cardiologic care of young women with NCCM is to inform patients that a pregnancy may carry a risk for themselves as well as for their offspring. For women with NCCM, the maternal risk in pregnancy for developing heart failure and/or arrhythmias requires extensive follow-up during pregnancies. Women with a cardiomyopathy who have symptoms before pregnancy have an increased risk and need specialized obstetric care [41]. Women with asymptomatic cardiomyopathies usually tolerate pregnancy well and these women may have a spontaneous labor and vaginal delivery [42]. NCCM patients have an increased risk of having a child with a cardiomyopathy. Depending on whether the patient has a mutation and the estimated risk for the child, prenatal diagnosis of NCCM (prenatal DNA testing and/or prenatal cardiac ultrasound of the fetus) can be discussed. Prenatal diagnostics for NCCM, however, are rarely requested, because the risk that a child has severe congenital NCCM is small, given that onset of symptoms of NCCM are age related, and patients/ carriers of mutations may not have symptoms. Unless there is an affected child in the family, in which case prenatal diagnostics for NCCM will be recommended.

The individual options and limitations of prenatal diagnosis of NCCM are discussed with NCCM patients with reproductive wishes. Pre- and post-test counseling is necessary because risks and prenatal testing in these pregnancies may evoke anxiety in parents and they may need help to make far reaching decisions during the pregnancy. It is important to acknowledge, that the likelihood that testing may cause distress, meaning that steps should be taken to minimize distress and provide support, not that testing should be denied.

For prenatal testing for NCCM the familial mutation is important. In families with a mutation, prenatal DNA testing can be performed. We have the choice of a DNA testing in chorionic villus sampling (conducted at 10–12 weeks of gestation) or amniocentesis (conducted at 14–20 weeks of gestation). The DNA test results are known within 2–3 weeks, well within the legal framework in most countries for terminating a pregnancy affected with a severe disorder. The parents need to be informed that these interventions carry a risk for the mother and fetus including miscarriage [43]. If the child is shown to have the familial mutation that may causes (severe) childhood cardiomyopathy, parents may choose to terminate the pregnancy or have additional prenatal echocardiography for structural defects and assessment of cardiac function to detect a congenital cardiomyopathy [44]. Prenatal cardiac sonography is performed in specialized tertiary prenatal centers, and allows to detect fetal cardiac malformations, cardiomyopathies, systolic and diastolic function and arrhythmia in the second –and third trimester of pregnancy. Prenatal cardiac sonography is also the method of choice for prenatal screening of NCCM when there is no mutation in the family. A major limitation of prenatal sonography for NCCM is that little is known about the onset and prenatal development of NCCM, and we do not know in which NCCM patients we may and in which we cannot find prenatally signs of noncompaction and in which trimester the first cardiac signs of noncompaction be may observed. There are few reports, showing early prenatal onset of NCCM in cases with a *MYH7* mutation [45]. Since prenatal diagnosed NCCM may remain asymptomatic after birth, prediction of disease severity from the results of prenatal testing remains difficult [46]. However, prenatal testing does have a role in assessment which pregnancy may need perinatal cardiac monitoring.

Psychological Impact of Genetic Testing for Index and for Relatives

Having a genetic cardiomyopathy implies that your children and other family members may have an increased risk of having a cardiomyopathy. For patients, this knowledge may add to the burden of having a cardiomyopathy. For insight in the psychological effects of genetic testing, we depend on studies focusing on familial cardiomyopathies or other genetic disorders. The studies looking at the impact of having a genetic cardiomyopathy showed that overall the burden of cardiac symptoms had greater psychosocial impact than the burden of the condition being genetic [26, 47]. Index cases might be pressured by their relatives to have genetic testing. But this did not negatively affect satisfaction with the genetic counseling process or getting the results of DNA testing [48]. Overall clinical symptoms are the principal source of concern: index cases showed more distress when having a diagnostic DNA test than relatives having a predictive DNA test, probably because the index cases had a cardiomyopathy, while the relatives usually are asymptomatic [49]. Predictive testing can evoke anxiety about risk of being affected and transmitting the predisposition for disease to offspring, but it may also bring clarity about a subject that has been on the mind for a significant time. Overall relatives at risk for hereditary cardiac diseases did not have more emotional distress the normal population [50]. Understandably, relatives with a positive genetic test showed more distress than relatives where a familial mutation could be excluded [49]. Despite the result of the genetic test, the vast majority (80%) of the patients was satisfied with the decision of undergoing a genetic test [49]. Patients who had less understanding of carriership of the mutation or had stronger belief in serious consequences had more symptoms of depression [47]. High levels of anxiety were linked to a younger age, females, less formal education and fewer social contacts [47, 51]. From these studies we have learned the importance of focusing during pre- and post-test counseling on the individual perception of risk and disease and helping the patients to cope with the consequences of the test result. The way of giving the test result, by telephone or by a face to face appointment, did not have an impact on contentment of the patient [48].

Cardiologic Screening

In case a mutation is identified in a patient, the patient is referred for cardiologic screening. Cardiologic screening is also recommended for relatives from a family with a mutation, who chooses not to have a predictive DNA test. Likewise, in families were no mutation is found, relatives are advised to have a cardiologic examination from age of 10 years onwards. Cardiologic screening may be initiated before the age of 10 years if the child is planning to engage in competitive sports, or there is a family history of sudden cardiac death. Cardiologic screening in family members contains a physical examination, 12-lead electrocardiography and echocardiography. When abnormalities are found the cardiac work up should be expanded. For example when signs of a cardiomyopathy on echocardiography are identified, additionally cardiac magnetic resonance imaging (CMR) can be performed. A48-h ambulatory electrocardiography should be performed when patients have palpitations or there are other indications for an arrhythmia.

In familial NCCM, relatives have less severe cardiac features than the index cases. Early detection in relatives is important and allows treatment and prevention of severe complications. Index cases with a mutation had a higher prevalence of familial disease. Cardiologic family screening is recommended for the families of all cases, because family screening may identify asymptomatic relatives with a cardiomyopathy in families without evidence for genetic disease. In this way cardiologic family screening may help to identify familial NCCM and stratify risk for relatives into a high genetic risk. In the sporadic cases without a mutation and negative results of cardiac family screening, as expected in approximately 50% of all cases diagnosed with NCCM, secondary causes (non-genetic) for NCCM are expected with low recurrence risks for relatives.

Cardiologic Follow-Up

In general, the diagnosis NCCM requires lifelong follow-up to detect changes in symptoms, risk for adverse events, LV function and cardiac rhythm. Prevalence of LV systolic dysfunction and atrial arrhythmias increases with age [52, 53]. The frequency of monitoring is determined by the severity of disease, age and symptoms. A clinical examination, including 12-lead ECG and TTE, should be performed every 1–2 years or sooner if patients have new cardiac symptoms [38]. In 50–70%

of the mutation carriers a cardiomyopathy is identified by first screening, 30% of these patients are asymptomatic [28, 54]. These asymptomatic carriers with a phenotype should also have follow-up every 1–2 years. The clinical significance of mild morphological and functional abnormalities is uncertain but probably minor in most [54, 55]. In 30% of the adult relatives with a mutation no cardiomyopathy at first cardiologic screening is identified, these are mutation carriers without a phenotype [28]. Studies suggest a benign clinical course for mutation carriers without a phenotype in HCM families [56, 57]. However, a proportion of mutation carriers without a phenotype will develop a cardiomyopathy later in life, because of age-related increase in penetrance [13]. This is why mutation carriers without a phenotype should have cardiac examination at least every 5 years [38]. Also first degree family members without a phenotype from families without a mutation cannot be discharged from medical follow-up and should also be screened at least every 5 years [38]. This is because not all genetic causes for NCCM are identified yet, and these relatives might have a yet unknown genetic cause for NCCM.

Genotype-Phenotype Correlation

Knowledge of the genetic cause for familial NCCM may help to predict the outcome. Specific genetic defects were associated with the phenotype, and associated clinical features, including risk for major adverse cardiac events for the index case and affected relatives. In other words, complementing cardiologic diagnosis with genetic status may allow tailoring clinical management and follow-up of familial NCCM according to genetic burden. In the future the associations between specific mutations and clinical features or risks may become clearer, by more extended methods of DNA testing and the analysis of the features large numbers of patients. Although specific genotype based cardiomyopathy treatments are not available, the established genotype-phenotype correlations for NCCM can help to guide clinical management of the patients.

Genetic Versus Sporadic NCCM

There are distinct differences between the genetic (the NCCM patients with a mutation and/or patients with a family history of cardiomyopathy) and the patients without a mutation or family history, the sporadic cases. Mutations occur more frequently in young patients and in patients with familial cardiomyopathies [4]. In children with genetic NCCM severe outcome of NCCM is more than in children with sporadic NCCM [4]. Children diagnosed before the age of 1 year, had frequently a mutation, cardiac symptoms, LV systolic dysfunction, and a high risk for major adverse cardiac events (MACE). In contrast to sporadic children, who had a good prognosis, with a mild clinical course and low risk for complications. In severe forms of NCCM occurring in childhood the possibility exists that it may involve a complex genotype. For that reason if a child is diagnosed with a cardiomyopathy in the family of an adult NCCM case, we recommend to perform a full panel of genes testing instead of only testing for the familial mutation.

Adults with a mutation had high risk for LV and RV systolic dysfunction [4]. Prognosis in adult NCCM patients with a mutation was correlated with left ventricular function. Adult NCCM patients with a mutation and a persevered LV ejection fraction had a good prognosis. In contrast to adults with a mutation and LV systolic dysfunction, who had worse outcome. In sporadic adult patients prognosis was not related to LV systolic function. The sporadic NCCM patients had frequently hypertension, suggesting an acquired form of NCCM, and this may have consequences for recommendations of family screening.

Sarcomere Genes

MYH7 gene mutations are the most prevalent genetic cause for NCCM are associated with a relatively milder course of disease with low risk for complications, compared to other genetic causes [4]. The prognosis for patients with mutations in the head of the *MYH7* gene was better than for patients with mutations in the tail of the gene [28]. Mutations in the head of *MYH7* were associated with NCCM with normal dimensions of the LV and a milder course of the disease. Mutations in the tail had high incidence of LV dilatation and LV systolic dysfunction. An explanation for the association between mutations in the tail and the dilated subtype could be that tail mutations may infer with the binding site for *TTN*, and thus may have a similar effect as the effect of *TTN* mutations, which are important causes of DCM. Also frequent relatives with DCM without hypertrabeculation were identified. Another feature of the *MYH7* was that this is one of the rare sarcomere genes that was observed in families where Ebstein anomaly occurred in NCCM patients [35]. The *TTN* gene, which is a major cause of DCM, is also a frequent cause of NCCM, predominantly in adult NCCM patients [4]. This could indicate that younger *TTN* carriers are not symptomatic, which may be important for relatives (children) who are carriers of a *TTN* mutation. The adult NCCM patients with *TTN* mutations had high prevalence of LV systolic dysfunction and LV dilatation, similar to DCM patients with *TTN* mutations. In families of NCCM patients with a *TTN* mutation relatives may have DCM without hypertrabeculation [28]. *MYBPC3* (compound) homozygous mutations were observed in NCCM cases with a severe phenotype and major cardiac events at young age [16]. NCCM patients with a single *MYBPC3* mutation had high prevalence of RV systolic dysfunction [4]. In the families of NCCM patients with a *MYBPC3* mutation, HCM without signs of hypertrabeculation may occur in relatives. Also an increased risk for LV hypertrophy (HCM) was observed [28]. Relatives with HCM without sigs of hypertrabeculation occur in the families of NCCM patients with a *MYBPC3* mutation.

Other Cardiomyopathy Genes

Mutations in *HCN4* were associated with NCCM and also bradycardia [58]. Mutations in *RYR2* lead to catecholaminergic polymorphic ventricular tachycardia (CPVT) and may also cause NCCM, especially variants in exon 3 [59]. *LMNA* and

RBM20 are rare causes for NCCM and may be associated with worse outcome, like in DCM [5]. *SCN5A* was reported to be a genetic modifier, increasing the risk for arrhythmias in NCCM [60].

Future Directions of Genetic Diagnosis and Family Screening for NCCM

The application of whole exome or genome sequencing of NCCM patients in the near future will reveal novel genetic causes or genetic interactions with modifiers, some of which may explain remodeling into different cardiomyopathy phenotypes within families. A disease model may be developed to obtain functional evidence of the deleterious effect of genetic variants for better understanding and a more accurate classification of the DNA variants in cardiomyopathy genes, especially for the variants that are now regarded as variants of unknown significance. The expected broad application in the general population of predictive DNA testing for genetic susceptibilities for a large range of disease, may achieve a change in attitude towards and the perception of having a genetic susceptibility. Because it is clear that all of us are carrying genetic defects for one disease or another. This awareness hopefully leads to ban the discriminatory socio economic sanctions experienced currently whenrevealing personal genetic burden.

Prospective large follow up studies are needed to confirm the genotype-phenotype correlations in NCCM, and adjust guidelines for clinical follow up of patients and at risk relatives accordingly. Leading eventually to family- and gene tailored follow-up and management of NCCM patients and their families. The risk for cardiomyopathy for relatives of sporadic NCCM patients seems low, also risk for mutation carriers without a phenotype seems low. Follow-up studies of these relatives at low risk are needed to evaluate the value of interval screening in these groups and to confirm the low risk. When al NCCM genes are known, excluding a genetic predisposition in a proportion of patients may be achieved, thus allowing making the important distinction between genetic and non-genetic NCCM. And follow-up strategies can be designed according to genetic burden. In the distant future genetic classification may lead to the development of genotype specific treatment and eventually gene therapy for NCCM.

Acknowledgement   J.I. van Waning is supported by a grant from the Jaap Schouten Foundation.

References

1. Bleyl SB, Mumford BR, Thompson V, Carey JC, Pysher TJ, Chin TK, et al. Neonatal, lethal noncompaction of the left ventricular myocardium is allelic with Barth Syndrome. Am J Hum Genet. 1997;61(4):868–72.
2. Hoedemaekers YM, Caliskan K, Majoor-Krakauer D, van de Laar I, Michels M, Witsenburg M, et al. Cardiac beta-myosin heavy chain defects in two families with non-compaction cardiomyopathy: linking non-compaction to hypertrophic, restrictive, and dilated cardiomyopathies. Eur Heart J. 2007;28(22):2732–7.

3. Klaassen S, Probst S, Oechslin E, Gerull B, Krings G, Schuler P, et al. Mutations in sarcomere protein genes in left ventricular noncompaction. Circulation. 2008;117(22):2893–901.
4. van Waning JI, Caliskan K, Hoedemaekers YM, van Spaendonck-Zwarts KY, Baas AF, Boekholdt SM, et al. Genetics, clinical features, and long-term outcome of noncompaction cardiomyopathy. J Am Coll Cardiol. 2018;71(7):711–22.
5. Sedaghat-Hamedani F, Haas J, Zhu F, Geier C, Kayvanpour E, Liss M, et al. Clinical genetics and outcome of left ventricular non-compaction cardiomyopathy. Eur Heart J. 2017;38(46):3449–60.
6. Charron P, Arad M, Arbustini E, Basso C, Bilinska Z, Elliott P, et al. Genetic counselling and testing in cardiomyopathies: a position statement of the European Society of Cardiology Working Group on Myocardial and Pericardial Diseases. Eur Heart J. 2010;31(22):2715–26.
7. Gati S, Rajani R, Carr-White GS, Chambers JB. Adult left ventricular noncompaction: reappraisal of current diagnostic imaging modalities. JACC Cardiovasc Imaging. 2014;7(12):1266–75.
8. Hoedemaekers YM, Caliskan K, Michels M, Frohn-Mulder I, van der Smagt JJ, Phefferkorn JE, et al. The importance of genetic counseling, DNA diagnostics, and cardiologic family screening in left ventricular noncompaction cardiomyopathy. Circ Cardiovasc Genet. 2010;3(3):232–9.
9. Kawel-Boehm N, McClelland RL, Zemrak F, Captur G, Hundley WG, Liu CY, et al. Hypertrabeculated left ventricular myocardium in relationship to myocardial function and fibrosis: the multi-ethnic study of atherosclerosis. Radiology. 2017;284:667.
10. Luijkx T, Cramer MJ, Zaidi A, Rienks R, Senden PJ, Sharma S, et al. Ethnic differences in ventricular hypertrabeculation on cardiac MRI in elite football players. Neth Heart J. 2012;20(10):389–95.
11. Gati S, Chandra N, Bennett RL, Reed M, Kervio G, Panoulas VF, et al. Increased left ventricular trabeculation in highly trained athletes: do we need more stringent criteria for the diagnosis of left ventricular non-compaction in athletes? Heart. 2013;99(6):401–8.
12. Vatta M, Mohapatra B, Jimenez S, Sanchez X, Faulkner G, Perles Z, et al. Mutations in Cypher/ZASP in patients with dilated cardiomyopathy and left ventricular non-compaction. J Am Coll Cardiol. 2003;42(11):2014–27.
13. Michels M, Soliman OI, Phefferkorn J, Hoedemaekers YM, Kofflard MJ, Dooijes D, et al. Disease penetrance and risk stratification for sudden cardiac death in asymptomatic hypertrophic cardiomyopathy mutation carriers. Eur Heart J. 2009;30(21):2593–8.
14. Budde BS, Binner P, Waldmuller S, Hohne W, Blankenfeldt W, Hassfeld S, et al. Noncompaction of the ventricular myocardium is associated with a de novo mutation in the beta-myosin heavy chain gene. PLoS One. 2007;2(12):e1362.
15. Maron BJ, Gardin JM, Flack JM, Gidding SS, Kurosaki TT, Bild DE. Prevalence of hypertrophic cardiomyopathy in a general population of young adults. Echocardiographic analysis of 4111 subjects in the CARDIA Study. Coronary Artery Risk Development in (Young) Adults. Circulation. 1995;92(4):785–9.
16. Wessels MW, Herkert JC, Frohn-Mulder IM, Dalinghaus M, van den Wijngaard A, de Krijger RR, et al. Compound heterozygous or homozygous truncating MYBPC3 mutations cause lethal cardiomyopathy with features of noncompaction and septal defects. Eur J Hum Genet. 2015;23(7):922–8.
17. Finsterer J, Stollberger C. Spontaneous left ventricular hypertrabeculation in dystrophin duplication based Becker's muscular dystrophy. Herz. 2001;26(7):477–81.
18. Amiya E, Morita H, Hatano M, Nitta D, Hosoya Y, Maki H, et al. Fukutin gene mutations that cause left ventricular noncompaction. Int J Cardiol. 2016;222:727–9.
19. Alston CL, Ceccatelli Berti C, Blakely EL, Olahova M, He L, McMahon CJ, et al. A recessive homozygous p.Asp92Gly SDHD mutation causes prenatal cardiomyopathy and a severe mitochondrial complex II deficiency. Hum Genet. 2015;134(8):869–79.
20. Finsterer J, Bittner R, Bodingbauer M, Eichberger H, Stollberger C, Blazek G. Complex mitochondriopathy associated with 4 mtDNA transitions. Eur Neurol. 2000;44(1):37–41.
21. Tang S, Batra A, Zhang Y, Ebenroth ES, Huang TS. Left ventricular noncompaction is associated with mutations in the mitochondrial genome. Mitochondrion. 2010;10(4):350–7.

22. Ojala T, Polinati P, Manninen T, Hiippala A, Rajantie J, Karikoski R, et al. New mutation of mitochondrial DNAJC19 causing dilated and noncompaction cardiomyopathy, anemia, ataxia, and male genital anomalies. Pediatr Res. 2012;72(4):432–7.
23. Cremer K, Ludecke HJ, Ruhr F, Wieczorek D. Left-ventricular non-compaction (LVNC): a clinical feature more often observed in terminal deletion 1p36 than previously expected. Eur J Med Genet. 2008;51(6):685–8.
24. Pauli RM, Scheib-Wixted S, Cripe L, Izumo S, Sekhon GS. Ventricular noncompaction and distal chromosome 5q deletion. Am J Med Genet. 1999;85(4):419–23.
25. McMahon CJ, Chang AC, Pignatelli RH, Miller-Hance WC, Eble BK, Towbin JA, et al. Left ventricular noncompaction cardiomyopathy in association with trisomy 13. Pediatr Cardiol. 2005;26(4):477–9.
26. Brouwers C, Caliskan K, Bos S, Van Lennep JE, Sijbrands EJ, Kop WJ, et al. Health status and psychological distress in patients with non-compaction cardiomyopathy: the role of burden related to symptoms and genetic vulnerability. Int J Behav Med. 2015;22(6):717–25.
27. Morales A, Cowan J, Dagua J, Hershberger RE. Family history: an essential tool for cardiovascular genetic medicine. Congest Heart Fail. 2008;14(1):37–45.
28. van Waning JI, Caliskan K, Michels M, Schinkel AFL, Hirsch A, Dalinghaus M, Hoedemaekers YM, Wessels MW, IJpma AS, Hofstra RMW, van Slegtenhorst MA, Majoor-Krakauer D. Cardiac phenotypes, genetics, and risks in familial noncompaction cardiomyopathy. J Am Coll Cardiol. 2019;73(13):1601–11. https://doi.org/10.1016/j.jacc.2018.12.085.
29. Plon SE, Eccles DM, Easton D, Foulkes WD, Genuardi M, Greenblatt MS, et al. Sequence variant classification and reporting: recommendations for improving the interpretation of cancer susceptibility genetic test results. Hum Mutat. 2008;29(11):1282–91.
30. Richards S, Aziz N, Bale S, Bick D, Das S, Gastier-Foster J, et al. Standards and guidelines for the interpretation of sequence variants: a joint consensus recommendation of the American College of Medical Genetics and Genomics and the Association for Molecular Pathology. Genet Med. 2015;17(5):405–24.
31. Abbasi Y, Jabbari J, Jabbari R, Yang RQ, Risgaard B, Kober L, et al. The pathogenicity of genetic variants previously associated with left ventricular non-compaction. Mol Genet Genomic Med. 2016;4(2):135–42.
32. Walsh R, Buchan R, Wilk A, John S, Felkin LE, Thomson KL, et al. Defining the genetic architecture of hypertrophic cardiomyopathy: re-evaluating the role of non-sarcomeric genes. Eur Heart J. 2017;38(46):3461–8.
33. Walsh R, Thomson KL, Ware JS, Funke BH, Woodley J, McGuire KJ, et al. Reassessment of Mendelian gene pathogenicity using 7,855 cardiomyopathy cases and 60,706 reference samples. Genet Med. 2017;19(2):192–203.
34. Stahli BE, Gebhard C, Biaggi P, Klaassen S, Valsangiacomo Buechel E, Attenhofer Jost CH, et al. Left ventricular non-compaction: prevalence in congenital heart disease. Int J Cardiol. 2013;167(6):2477–81.
35. Vermeer AM, van Engelen K, Postma AV, Baars MJ, Christiaans I, De Haij S, et al. Ebstein anomaly associated with left ventricular noncompaction: an autosomal dominant condition that can be caused by mutations in MYH7. Am J Med Genet C Semin Med Genet. 2013;163C(3):178–84.
36. Ichida F, Tsubata S, Bowles KR, Haneda N, Uese K, Miyawaki T, et al. Novel gene mutations in patients with left ventricular noncompaction or Barth syndrome. Circulation. 2001;103(9):1256–63.
37. van der Roest WP, Pennings JM, Bakker M, van den Berg MP, van Tintelen JP. Family letters are an effective way to inform relatives about inherited cardiac disease. Am J Med Genet A. 2009;149A(3):357–63.
38. Authors/Task Force Members, Elliott PM, Anastasakis A, Borger MA, Borggrefe M, Cecchi F, et al. 2014 ESC guidelines on diagnosis and management of hypertrophic cardiomyopathy: the Task Force for the Diagnosis and Management of Hypertrophic Cardiomyopathy of the European Society of Cardiology (ESC). Eur Heart J. 2014;35(39):2733–79.
39. Fanos JH. Developmental tasks of childhood and adolescence: implications for genetic testing. Am J Med Genet. 1997;71(1):22–8.

40. Bratt EL, Ostman-Smith I, Axelsson A, Berntsson L. Quality of life in asymptomatic children and adolescents before and after diagnosis of hypertrophic cardiomyopathy through family screening. J Clin Nurs. 2013;22(1–2):211–21.
41. Pieper PG, Walker F. Pregnancy in women with hypertrophic cardiomyopathy. Neth Heart J. 2013;21(1):14–8.
42. European Society of Gynecology, Association for European Paediatric Cardiology, German Society for Gender Medicine, Regitz-Zagrosek V, Blomstrom Lundqvist C, Borghi C, et al. ESC guidelines on the management of cardiovascular diseases during pregnancy: the Task Force on the Management of Cardiovascular Diseases during Pregnancy of the European Society of Cardiology (ESC). Eur Heart J. 2011;32(24):3147–97.
43. Tabor A, Philip J, Madsen M, Bang J, Obel EB, Norgaard-Pedersen B. Randomised controlled trial of genetic amniocentesis in 4606 low-risk women. Lancet. 1986;1(8493):1287–93.
44. Pedra SR, Smallhorn JF, Ryan G, Chitayat D, Taylor GP, Khan R, et al. Fetal cardiomyopathies: pathogenic mechanisms, hemodynamic findings, and clinical outcome. Circulation. 2002;106(5):585–91.
45. Hoedemaekers YM, Cohen-Overbeek TE, Frohn-Mulder IM, Dooijes D, Majoor-Krakauer DF. Prenatal ultrasound diagnosis of MYH7 non-compaction cardiomyopathy. Ultrasound Obstet Gynecol. 2013;41(3):336–9.
46. Stollberger C, Wegner C, Benatar A, Chin TK, Dangel J, Majoor-Krakauer D, et al. Postnatal outcome of fetal left ventricular hypertrabeculation/noncompaction. Pediatr Cardiol. 2016;37(5):919–24.
47. Christiaans I, van Langen IM, Birnie E, Bonsel GJ, Wilde AA, Smets EM. Quality of life and psychological distress in hypertrophic cardiomyopathy mutation carriers: a cross-sectional cohort study. Am J Med Genet A. 2009;149A(4):602–12.
48. Christiaans I, van Langen IM, Birnie E, Bonsel GJ, Wilde AA, Smets EM. Genetic counseling and cardiac care in predictively tested hypertrophic cardiomyopathy mutation carriers: the patients' perspective. Am J Med Genet A. 2009;149A(7):1444–51.
49. Wynn J, Holland DT, Duong J, Ahimaz P, Chung WK. Examining the psychosocial impact of genetic testing for cardiomyopathies. J Genet Couns. 2018;27:927.
50. Hoedemaekers E, Jaspers JP, Van Tintelen JP. The influence of coping styles and perceived control on emotional distress in persons at risk for a hereditary heart disease. Am J Med Genet A. 2007;143A(17):1997–2005.
51. Vernon SW, Gritz ER, Peterson SK, Amos CI, Baile WF, Perz CA, et al. Design and methodology of a study of psychosocial aspects of genetic testing for hereditary colorectal cancer. Ann N Y Acad Sci. 1997;833:190–4.
52. Olivotto I, Cecchi F, Casey SA, Dolara A, Traverse JH, Maron BJ. Impact of atrial fibrillation on the clinical course of hypertrophic cardiomyopathy. Circulation. 2001;104(21):2517–24.
53. Thaman R, Gimeno JR, Murphy RT, Kubo T, Sachdev B, Mogensen J, et al. Prevalence and clinical significance of systolic impairment in hypertrophic cardiomyopathy. Heart. 2005;91(7):920–5.
54. Charron P, Dubourg O, Desnos M, Bouhour JB, Isnard R, Hagege A, et al. Diagnostic value of electrocardiography and echocardiography for familial hypertrophic cardiomyopathy in genotyped children. Eur Heart J. 1998;19(9):1377–82.
55. Gandjbakhch E, Gackowski A, Tezenas du Montcel S, Isnard R, Hamroun A, Richard P, et al. Early identification of mutation carriers in familial hypertrophic cardiomyopathy by combined echocardiography and tissue Doppler imaging. Eur Heart J. 2010;31(13):1599–607.
56. Jensen MK, Havndrup O, Christiansen M, Andersen PS, Diness B, Axelsson A, et al. Penetrance of hypertrophic cardiomyopathy in children and adolescents: a 12-year follow-up study of clinical screening and predictive genetic testing. Circulation. 2013;127(1):48–54.
57. Gray B, Ingles J, Semsarian C. Natural history of genotype positive-phenotype negative patients with hypertrophic cardiomyopathy. Int J Cardiol. 2011;152(2):258–9.
58. Milano A, Vermeer AM, Lodder EM, Barc J, Verkerk AO, Postma AV, et al. HCN4 mutations in multiple families with bradycardia and left ventricular noncompaction cardiomyopathy. J Am Coll Cardiol. 2014;64(8):745–56.

59. Campbell MJ, Czosek RJ, Hinton RB, Miller EM. Exon 3 deletion of ryanodine receptor causes left ventricular noncompaction, worsening catecholaminergic polymorphic ventricular tachycardia, and sudden cardiac arrest. Am J Med Genet A. 2015;167A(9):2197–200.
60. Shan L, Makita N, Xing Y, Watanabe S, Futatani T, Ye F, et al. SCN5A variants in Japanese patients with left ventricular noncompaction and arrhythmia. Mol Genet Metab. 2008;93(4):468–74.

Long-term Prognosis and Management of Noncompaction Cardiomyopathy

9

Emrah Kaya, Martijn Otten, and Kadir Caliskan

Introduction

Currently NCCM is viewed as a primary cardiomyopathy, with mostly autosomal dominant inheritance pattern [1]. The clinical presentation varies from asymptomatic to supra-ventricular arrhythmias, severe heart failure (HF), malignant ventricular arrhythmias, and thromboembolic events [2, 3]. Since the first report by Engberding and Bender in 1984 of a case of a 33 years old women with heart failure and palpitations and later in 1990 case series of 8 patients by Chin et al., there is increasing amounts of publications and more awareness among clinicians. But the majority of these are small series of cases or solely case reports with high incidence of adverse cardiac events, probably reflecting the biased patient selection in tertiary referral centers. Therefore, the long-term prognosis remains conflicting and inconsistent. In this chapter, we report our single center experience with excellent long-term survival in patients without heart failure in the modern heart failure treatment area with individualized drug treatment and, in selected patients, ICD implantation for primary or secondary prophylaxes of sudden cardiac death [4, 5]. We also provide an overview of the most up-to-date prognosis studies. Noncompaction cardiomyopathy remains yet a relative rare, primary cardiomyopathy with potentially grave prognosis in different case series [2, 6, 7]. Major causes of mortality and morbidity are due to trias of heart

E. Kaya
Thoraxcenter, Department of Cardiology, Erasmus MC University Medical Center, Rotterdam, The Netherlands

Department of Cardiology, Onze Lieve Vrouwe Gasthuis, Amsterdam, The Netherlands

M. Otten
Thoraxcenter, Department of Cardiology, Erasmus MC University Medical Center, Rotterdam, The Netherlands

K. Caliskan (✉)
Erasmus MC University Medical Center, Department of Cardiology, Rotterdam, The Netherlands
e-mail: k.caliskan@erasmusmc.nl

© Springer Nature Switzerland AG 2019   149
K. Caliskan et al. (eds.), *Noncompaction Cardiomyopathy*,
https://doi.org/10.1007/978-3-030-17720-1_9

failure, sudden cardiac death and/or thrombo-embolic events [8]. The first case series reported a very high risk of mortality and morbidity, although the recent reports are far more favorable and benign short- and midterm prognosis [3, 9]. In a report with 2.3 years of follow-up, there was a high incidence (66%) of severe outcome, including cardiac transplantation, death, hospitalizations for heart failure or severe rhythm disorders [10]. Importantly, these poor outcomes were largely related to symptomatic patients with heart failure symptoms and signs. In another study with a median follow-up time of 2.7 years, none of the asymptomatic patients died or needed cardiac transplantation compared to 31% of the symptomatic patients [11]. Outcomes and phenotypes may differ between children and adults. Nationwide survey in Japan over 20 years of patients with NCCM confirmed the poor prognosis for both infantile and juvenile types, were heart failure and hypoplasia of the compacted layer of the left ventricular wall are the major factors of poor prognosis [12, 13]. Therefore ongoing follow-up is recommended in all NCCM patients.

Natural History

In 1984, Engberding and Bender described a 33 years old patient with persistent myocardial sinusoids as a rare congenital anomaly [14]. Six years later, Chin et al. published a series of 8 pediatric and adolescent patients with increased trabeculation of the left ventricular (LV) endocardium and described isolated noncompaction of left ventricular myocardium as a separate disease entity [15].

The largest series to date for NCCM patients are small but comprehend the most information related to the natural history of NCCM [2, 6, 7, 15, 16]. The natural history of NCCM is variable and symptoms may develop during all phases of life, from childhood to old age [14].

NCCM typically presents with normal left ventricle size, systolic- and diastolic function, or as a primary dilated cardiomyopathy with or without restrictive left ventricular hemodynamics [8]. Despite the lack of longitudinal studies in adults with NCCM, most patients diagnosed in childhood will develop systolic dysfunction of the left ventricle after a follow-up period longer than 10 years [6]. In a recent retrospectively study (reviewed between 2008–2014) there were 62 patients identified with NCCM. The patients with LVEF ≤40% were older (67 vs 54 years; P = 0.006), had more congestive heart failure (72% vs 21%; P < 0.001) and hypertension (83% vs 52%; P = 0.01) and significant QRS interval prolongation [17]. Earlier reports have shown that a QRS duration >120 ms, as well as an absolute increase in QRS duration, are independent predictors of mortality in patients with NCCM [18].

A nationwide survey over two decades of NCCM patients revealed a poor prognosis for both infantile (diagnosed at <1 year of age: 108 cases) and juvenile types (diagnosed 1–15 years of age: 97 cases). Heart failure at diagnosis and hypoplasia of the compacted layer of the left ventricular wall are found to be the major determinants of poor prognosis. Therefore, ongoing follow up is recommended in adulthood [12].

According to another recent published study, in this heterogeneous cardiomyopathy, age at diagnosis, LV systolic dysfunction, and risk of MACE were related to genetic status. This study showed that nearly one-third of the NCCM patients had a mutation in a cardiomyopathy gene. In children with NCCM, the genetic cause is more common compared to adults. Systolic dysfunction of the left ventricle at presentation and long-term outcome were also linked to genetics [19]. This report emphasizes the importance of distinguishing genetic NCCM because genetic status may add to prediction of risk for major adverse cardiovascular event (MACE). It may also be helpful in clinical management and intensity of follow-up. Children with a mutation were often diagnosed under an age of 1 year. They demonstrated that these patients had cardiac symptoms, LV systolic dysfunction, and a high risk for MACE. However, children with sporadic NCCM (no mutation or family history of cardiomyopathy) were diagnosed incidentally, had normal cardiac function, and low risk of MACE. Adults with a mutation were strongly correlated with a high risk of MACE and LV systolic dysfunction. Although, risk of MACE in adults with sporadic NCCM (no mutation or family history of cardiomyopathy) wasn't determined by LV systolic dysfunction. In a recent comprehensive study by Van Waning & Caliskan et al. of Dutch patients with NCCM, Waning & Caliskan et al. describes that MYH7, MYBPC3, and TTN mutations were the most common mutations (71%) with higher rate of LV systolic dysfunction in patients with mutations vs probably familial and sporadic cases (p = 0.024). The highest risk of cardiovascular complications were in patients with multiple or TTN mutations. Same pattern was also seen in the pediatric patients, were mutation rate was much higher (p = 0.04) and associated with MACE (p = 0.025). Only the patients with MYH7 mutations had lower risk for MACE (p = 0.03). This study confirms that NCCM is a heterogeneous condition, and that genetic screening can have a important role in clinical stratification [19].

Long-Term Prognosis and Outcome

Non-compaction cardiomyopathy outcomes are to be viewed within specific subgroups of the disease rather than as non-compaction as a whole. Even patients that progress relatively discrete can be at risk for sudden death, congestive heart failure, atrium fibrillation and thromboembolic events [20]. Even though these events could occur in all NCCM patients, specific subgroups are at higher risk. Patients with heart failure at presentation, a very low age at presentation, a lower LVEF, arrhythmias (especially with malignant ventricular arrhythmias) and patients with a coexisting neuromuscular disease (NMD) have a higher mortality [9, 10, 19, 21–28].

Adult patients. Death/HTX rates reported in NCCM in adult populations range from 47% in a mean follow up of 3.6 years by Oechslin et al. described in 2000 to 15% in a mean follow of 6.6 years in a recent publication by Stämpfi et al. in 2017 [2, 24]. Most studies show a mortality rate of around 21% in a follow up of approximately 4.2 years. (Table 9.1) Most of this mortality is due to either sudden death or heart failure.

In a serie of Greutman et al. none of the asymptomatic patients died, while a death/HTX rate of 31% was found in symptomatic patients after a median follow up of 2.7 years [33]. Similarly Habib et al. and Lofiego et al. found patients with an incidental or familial detection to have a better prognosis than patients who presented with heart failure or ventricular dysfunction [10, 26]. These findings are confirmed in our experience when comparing patients with primary presentation with HF with

Table 9.1 Comparison of clinical features of adult patients in different cohort studies

	van Waning et al. (2018) [19]	Li [29]	Arenas et al. (2018) [17]	Stämpfli et al. (2017) [24]	Asfalou et al. (2017) [25]	Andreini et al. (2016) [30]	Stöllberger et al. (2015) [22]	Peters [31]	Kimura [32]	Tian et al. (2013) [21]	Greutmann et al. (2012) [33]	Habib et al. (2011) [10]	Caliskan et al. (2011) [5]	Correia (2011) [34]	Steffel et al. (2011) [23]	Lofiego et al. (2007) [26]	Aras (2006) [9]	Murphy et al. (2005) [3]	Oechslin et al. (2000) [2]	Pooled means[a]
Number of patients	194	83	62	153	23	113	220	55	35	106	132	105	77	20	74	65	67	45	34	1598
Male (%)	54	72	68	60	65	62	69	38	100	78	35	66	48	65	53	37	66	62	74	50 (±15)
Mean age (years)	45b	42	63	43	47	44	52	42	24	46	41	45	40	53	43	45	41	37	42	45 (±18)
NMD (%)	–	–	–	–	0	6	61	0	100	1	–	–	–	–	–	9	0	–	–	27 (±37) range
Family history (%)	36	6	–	–	4	15	–	–	–	11	23	18	43	10	–	31	33	51	18	26 (±14)
Presentation (%)																				
• Heart failure	26	–	56	–	51	–	–	–	–	–	33	57	43	35	34	62	–	–	62	42 (±13)
• Arrhythmias	34	–	11	–	17	–	–	–	–	–	21	15	32	30	22	9	–	–	6	24 (±25)
Thrombo-embolic event	3	–	10	–	4	–	–	–	–	–	5	7	12	10	8	–	–	–	–	6.4 (±3.2)
Screening	22	–	–	–	4	–	–	–	–	–	8	8	–	10	5	15	9	3	3	12 (±6.3)
LVEDD (mm)	–	61	56	–	68	–	60	59	51	64	34c	63	60	58	33c	67	58	58	65	60 (±11)
LVEF (%)	–	31.6	31	–	27	43	–	30	34	39	41	–	–	45	40	31	44	–	33	39 (±16)
NYHA class III or IV (%)	–	–	58	12	–	–	37	9	–	60	35	48	30	10	–	32	30	36	35	34 (±16)
LVEF moderate or severe (%)	–	–	69	–	–	–	–	–	–	–	–	–	–	30	–	–	–	–	–	59 (±28)
ICD (%)	–	–	24	–	17	–	–	2	0	10	–	28	57	15	–	17	1	4	12	20 (±18)
Mean follow-up (years)	2b	4.5b	3.5	6.6	2	4	6.0	1.3	3.2b	2.9	2.7b	2.3	2.8	1.0	4.5	4	2.5	3.8	3.6	3.7 (±1.4)
HTX (%)	2	5	–	5	0	–	–	–	–	4	5	8	3	5	0	14	0	0	12	4.2 (±4.5)

Total mortality (%)	6	27	15	10	17	4[d]	30	13	37	23	21	11	5	11	5	11	25	10	2	35	15 (±11)
HTX or mortality (%)	–	32	–	15	17	–	30	–	–	26	26	20	8	10	11	10	25	10	2	47	21 (±12)
Multivariate predictors of worse outcome	–	–	–	NYHA, LVEF, NT-proBNP, exercise capacity[e]	NYHA, LVEF, AF, male, LVEDD, BBB, >5 NC seg., NC/C > 2.2[f]	LGE[g]	NYHA, AF, NMD, age, tachycardia[f]	–	–	RBBB[c]	–	High LV fill, HF[e]	–	QTc, repolarisation ab. inf.[e]	–	NYHA, ven. Arr. LAD[e]	NYHA, LVEF[d]	–	NYHA, LVEF 3x, AF 2x, age, male, BBB, RBBB, LVEDD, NMD, LGE, >5 NC seg.. NC/C > 2.2, HF, tachycardia, high LV pres, QTc, repolarisation ab. inf. ven. Arr. NT-proBNP exercise capacity	–	NYHA 5x,

LVEDD left ventricle end diastolic diameter, *LVEF* left ventricle ejection fraction, *NYHA* New York Heart Association class, *ICD* Implantable Cardioverter Defibrillator, *NMD* neuromuscular disease, *HTX* heart transplantation, *HF* heart failure, *AF* atrium fibrillation, *R/L BBB* right/left bundle branch block, *LGE* late gadolinium enhancement, *seg.* segments, *NC/C* non compacted/compacted ratio, *fill.* filling pressure, *ab. inf.* Abnormalities in inferior lead, *ve. arr.* ventricular arrhythmia, *LAD* left atrium diameter, ± standard deviation

a Medians were seen as means for calculation only in calculation of SD for continues variables only medians were not used
b Median
c Indexed by body surface area
d Only cardiac death
e Combined endpoint of mortality or HTX
f Mortality only
g Cardiac mortality only

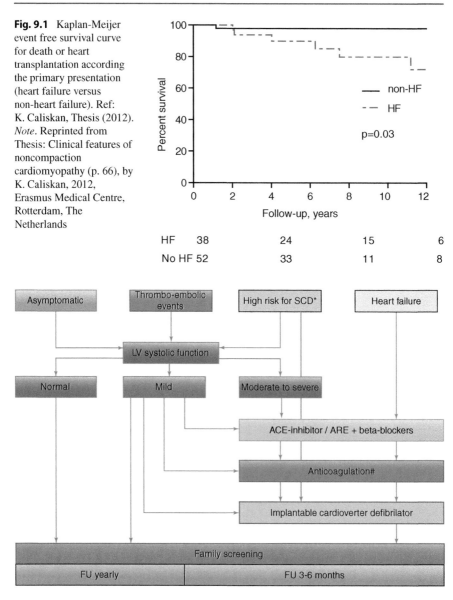

Fig. 9.1 Kaplan-Meijer event free survival curve for death or heart transplantation according the primary presentation (heart failure versus non-heart failure). Ref: K. Caliskan, Thesis (2012). *Note*. Reprinted from Thesis: Clinical features of noncompaction cardiomyopathy (p. 66), by K. Caliskan, 2012, Erasmus Medical Centre, Rotterdam, The Netherlands

Fig. 9.2 Strategy proposal for clinical management of patients with NCCM. *Note*. Adapted from Thesis: Clinical features of noncompaction cardiomyopathy (p. 68), by K. Caliskan, 2012, Erasmus Medical Centre, Rotterdam, The Netherlands

versus without HF (Fig. 9.1). A pattern of successive reports of poor and better prognosis is not unique to NCCM. Similarly, the first studies in hypertrophic cardiomyopathy reported a very poor prognosis with latter studies reporting a better outcome [36]. This is probably due to selection of the sickest patients for early referral to tertiary centers with subsequent referral of patients with milder symptoms and their

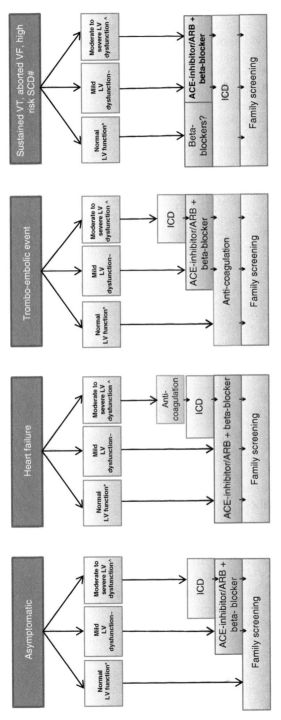

Fig. 9.3 Management of noncompaction cardiomyopathy patients according to the primary presentation. *Denotes ejection fraction >50%; ~ ejection fraction 40–50%; ^ ejection fration <40%, *VF* ventricle tachycardia, *VT* ventricle tachycardia. *VF* ventricle fibrillation, *LV* left ventricle, *ICD* implantable cardioverter-defibrillator, *ACE* angiotensin converting enzyme, *ARB* angiotensin receptor blocker; # high risk for sudden cardiac death: nonsustained VT's and on of the following risk factors: EF < 50%, family history of sudden cardiac <50 years, early repolarizations and/or fragmented QRS complexes (Guidelines HeartRhythm, AHA/ACC, ESC…)

asymptomatic relatives [37]. In NCCM, increasing knowledge among physicians and better imaging modalities also may explain this phenomenon.

Neuromuscular disease is reported to be associated with unfavorable outcomes in NCCM. In a cohort of Stöllberger et al. NMD is found as a predictor of mortality in multivariate analysis [22]. In line with their findings a study from Kimura et al. with a population of patients Duchenne or Becker muscular dystrophy and NCCM showed a 37% mortality in a median 3.2 years follow up. They also compared patients with these NMD with NCCM with patients with NCCM and found a significant lower survival in the NCCM group (Figs. 9.2 and 9.3).

Left ventricular ejection fraction (LVEF) is a strong predictor of worse outcomes. Aras et al. found that each 1% lower LVEF was associated with a 0.82 times increased mortality in multivariate analysis. Comparably Stämpfi et al. who found an adjusted HR of 2.68 (95% CI 1.62–4.41) for death/HTX. These findings are in line with univariate analysis in other long term cohort studies [2, 10, 21, 29, 30].

Pediatric patients. The prognosis of NCCM diagnosed in childhood differs from adults, as do some of the risk factors. An overview of the current available literature is shown in the Table 9.2. Death/HTX rates in children range from 7% in a median of 7 years to 52% in a median follow-up of 1.2 years [6, 27]. Notable, in this study with the low death/HTX rate, the majority (74%) of the patients had an asymptomatic presentation [6]. In the study with the high event rate, the patients were very young at diagnosis, median 0.3 years old [27]. In line with this report Shi et al. found in their population of median 0.3 years old at diagnosis a 69% death/HTX rate with a median follow up of 7 years [28]. A presentation under the age of 1 year is found to be a predictor in univariate analysis of worse outcome in three other studies [12, 19, 35]. Interestingly, in the study of Wang et al. infantile age at presentation was not found as a predictor of long term outcomes for a combined endpoint of death, HTX or ICD implantation in multivariate analysis.

Whereas mortality outcomes differ considerably more favorable outcomes are found in more recent studies. Among the studies that looked at risk factors are ECG abnormalities, but here no consistent line can be seen. Heart failure, a low LVEF, NMD, heart failure and arrhythmias on the other hand are more consistently found and show significant higher mortality/HTX risks. NCCM patients with these risk factors could benefit from more aggressive therapy.

Management of Noncompaction Cardiomyopathy

Currently, the management of NCCM patients are solely based on empirical treatment and clinical experience. The primary presentation, i.e. symptoms and signs at diagnosis combined with the severity of LV dysfunction, guides the appropriate drug and device treatment strategy. In patients with HF and/or significant LV dysfunction, treatment with beta-blockers, ACE-inhibitors and anticoagulants is appropriate. ICD implantation is appropriate in all patients presenting with sustained VT of VF and in selected patients with potentially high-risk features, including (unexplained) syncope, non-sustained VTs at Holter monitoring, early repolarization at surface electrocardiogram and/or a family history of premature sudden cardiac

Table 9.2 Comparison of clinical features of pediatric patients in different cohort studies

	van Waning et al. (2018) [19]	Tian (2018) [38]	Shi et al. (2018) [28]	Wang et al. (2017) [12]		Czosek (2015) [39]	Jefferies (2015) [40]	Brescia et al. (2013) [35]	Zuckerman et al. (2011) [27]	Çeliker (2005) [41]	Wald (2004) [42]	Ichida et al. (1999) [6]	Pouled means[a]
Number of patients	52	41	29	108	97	72	35	155	50	11	22	27	699
Male (%)	52	28	69	55	53	65	68	64	48	64	41	56	56 ± 12
Mean age (years)	7[b]	14	0.3[b]	0.2[b]	7.3[b]	13	8.1	4.7	0.3[b]	7.3	3.9	6	6.2(±7.4)
NMD (%)	–	5	24	–	–	–	–	–	14	–	14	–	13 (±7.7)
Family history (%)	40	10	31	37	36	–	6	23	–	18	36	52	30 (±14)
Presentation (%)													
Asymptomatic	17	76	–	21	52	–	–	–	–	27	14	74	39 (±29)
Congestive heart failure	31	24	83	65	22	–	41	25	–	36	55	26	31 (±20)
Arrhythmias	27	49	–	9	11	–	–	10	–	27	14	–	16 (±15)
Screening	17	–	–	–	–	–	–	14	–	–	–	–	15 (±2.1)
LVEDD (mm)	–	38[c]	–	–	–	–	–	–	–	–	53[b]	–	43 (± –)
LVEF (%)	–	41	–	43	57	–	–	–	–	52	34[b]	62	47 (±10)
NYHA class III or IV (%)	–	24	–	–	–	–	–	–	–	–	–	–	24 (± –)
LVEF moderate or severe (%)	42 <45%	–	–	–	–	0	–	–	–	27	–	48[d]	23 (±21)
ICD (%)	–	–	–	1	1	0	–	–	–	55	–	4	3.8 (±24)
Mean follow-up (years)	5[b]	2.9	7[b]	4.9[b]	–	Up to 4	3	4[b]	1.2[b]	3.5	3[b]	6[b]	4.2 (±1.5)
HTX (%)	8	5	21	5	4	0	12	5	30	0	9	0	7.2 (±9.1)
Total mortality (%)	16	5	48	13	9	1	14 on 5-year	13	22	27	13	7	13 (±12)

(continued)

Table 9.2 (continued)

	van Waning et al. (2018) [19]	Tian (2018) [38]	Shi et al. (2018) [28]	Wang et al. (2017) [12]	Czosek (2015) [39]	Jefferies (2015) [40]	Brescia et al. (2013) [35]	Zuckerman et al. (2011) [27]	Çeliker (2005) [41]	Wald (2004) [42]	Ichida et al. (1999) [6]	Pouled means[a]
HTX or mortality (%)	–	9	69	18	13	26	18	52	27	23	7	20 (±19)
Univariate predictors of worse outcome	Presentation <1year[e]	LVEF, HF, lower bp, LGE[f]	–	Presentation <1 year, LVEF, HF, LVPWC	–	Dilated phenotype[f]	Presentation <1 year, cardiac dys., T inv., ST seg. Ab., arr.[f]	FS, LVEDD, met/gen, H/D instability at presentation[f]	–	NC/C ratio[g]	–	Presentation <1 year 3x, LVEF 2x, HF 2x, LVPWC, LGE, lower bp, dilated phenotype, cardiac dysfunction, T wave inversion, ST seg ab. Arr. FS, LVEDD, met/gen, H/D instability at pres, N/C ratio

LVEDD left ventricle end diastolic diameter, *LVEF* left ventricle ejection fraction, *NYHA* New York Heart Association class, *ICD* Implantable Cardioverter Defibrillator, *NMD* neuromuscular disease, *HTX* heart transplantation, *HF* heart failure, *BP* blood pressure, *LGE* late gadolinium enhancement, *seg.* segments, *NC/C* non compacted/compacted ratio, *LVPWC* thickness of compacted layer in LV posterior wall, *dys.* dysfunction, *T inv.* T top inversion, *ST seg. ab.* ST segment abnormality, *arr.* arrhythmia, *FS* fractional shortening, *met/gen* associated metabolic and/or genetic syndrome, *H/D* hemodynamic, ± standard deviation

[a]Medians were seen as means for calculation only in calculation of SD for continues variables only medians were not used
[b]Median
[c]Indexed by body surface area
[d]Depressed at papillary level
[e]Mortality only
[f]Combined endpoint of mortality or HTX
[g]Combined endpoint of mortality or HTX or listing for HTX

death. Apart from sudden cardiac death, which may be prevented in part by timely implantation of an ICD, and LV dysfunction, which may be managed by appropriate drug therapy, patients with NCCM may develop intra-ventricular thrombosis and subsequent emboli. At a considerable long-term follow-up of our adult NCCM population, we observed in our center only two such cases, both in patients with moderate to severe impaired LV function. However, the majority of patients (84% in HF versus 50% in non HF patients) were already empirically treated with preventive anticoagulation. Thus a more liberal prescription of anticoagulants appears appropriate. Based on our observations and those from other patients series, we developed a treatment guideline for NCCM as shown in Table 9.2. The primary presentation, i.e. symptoms and signs at diagnosis, combined with the severity of LV dysfunction, guides the appropriate drug and device treatment strategy. In patients with HF and/ or significant LV dysfunction, treatment with beta-blockers, ACE-inhibitors and anticoagulants is appropriate. ICD implantation is appropriate in all patients presenting with sustained VT of VF and in selected patients with potentially high risk features, including (unexplained) syncope, non-sustained VTs at Holter monitoring, early repolarization at surface electrocardiogram and/or a family history of premature sudden cardiac death. Further evidence, to improve outcome in patients with this rare disease, could come from multicenter registry-based studies, similar to those in other cardiomyopathies [43, 44]. Furthermore, large case series remain an important source of information to develop an appropriate diagnostic strategy and to improve treatment of NCCM.

Conclusions and Feature Perspectives

The natural history of this disease and the long-term prognosis are still topic of discussion. The first case series reported a very high risk of mortality and morbidity, recent reports are far more favorable and benign short- and midterm prognosis. Studies show that patients with heart failure at presentation, an age <1 year at presentation, a lower LVEF, arrhythmias and patients with a coexisting neuromuscular disease (NMD) have a higher mortality. Most of this mortality is due to either sudden death or heart failure. Left ventricular ejection fraction (LVEF) is a strong predictor of worse outcomes. Patients without heart failure however, have excellent long-term (5 years) survival, fully comparable with the general population. In patients with HF and/or significant LV dysfunction, is however, prognosis clearly endangered and therefore, (prophylactic) treatment with beta-blockers, ACE-inhibitors and anticoagulants is inevitable. ICD implantation is appropriate in all patients presenting with sustained VT of VF and in selected patients with potentially high risk features, including (unexplained) syncope, non-sustained VTs at Holter monitoring, early repolarization at surface electrocardiogram and/or a family history of premature sudden cardiac death. More precise answers are required, based on pathologic, clinical, and genetic analyses. Prospective multicenter, international registries, and consensus statements like in other cardiomyopathies could aid to clarify current uncertainties. Due to the genetic heterogeneity and lack of clear view on the genotype-phenotype relationship of NCCM, further studies with comprehensive genetic counseling, DNA diagnostics, and cardiologic family screening should be conducted. Futhermore, prevention of SCD and therefore appropriate risk stratification remains highly challenging. Strategies to improve outcome of patients with this rare disease could be obtained by large multicenter registry-based studies.

References

1. Maron BJ, Towbin JA, Thiene G, Antzelevitch C, Corrado D, Arnett D, Moss AJ, Seidman CE, Young JB, American Heart Association, Council on Clinical Cardiology, Heart Failure and Transplantation Committee, Quality of Care and Outcomes Research and Functional Genomics and Translational Biology Interdisciplinary Working Groups, Council on Epidemiology and Prevention. Contemporary definitions and classification of the cardiomyopathies: an American Heart Association Scientific Statement from the Council on Clinical Cardiology, Heart Failure and Transplantation Committee; Quality of Care and Outcomes Research and Functional Genomics and Translational Biology Interdisciplinary Working Groups; and Council on Epidemiology and Prevention. Circulation. 2006;113:1807–16.
2. Oechslin EN, Attenhofer Jost CH, Rojas JR, Kaufmann PA, Jenni R. Long-term follow-up of 34 adults with isolated left ventricular noncompaction: a distinct cardiomyopathy with poor prognosis. J Am Coll Cardiol. 2000;36:493–500.
3. Murphy RT, Thaman R, Blanes JG, Ward D, Sevdalis E, Papra E, Kiotsekoglou A, Tome MT, Pellerin D, McKenna WJ, Elliott PM. Natural history and familial characteristics of isolated left ventricular non-compaction. Eur Heart J. 2005;26:187–92.
4. Heart Failure Society of America, Lindenfeld J, Albert NM, Boehmer JP, Collins SP, Ezekowitz JA, Givertz MM, Katz SD, Klapholz M, Moser DK, Rogers JG, Starling RC, Stevenson WG, Tang WH, Teerlink JR, Walsh MN. HFSA 2010 comprehensive heart failure practice guideline. J Card Fail. 2010;16:e1–194.
5. Caliskan K, Szili-Torok T, Theuns DA, Kardos A, Geleijnse ML, Balk AH, van Domburg RT, Jordaens L, Simoons ML. Indications and outcome of implantable cardioverter-defibrillators for primary and secondary prophylaxis in patients with noncompaction cardiomyopathy. J Cardiovasc Electrophysiol. 2011;22:898–904.
6. Ichida F, Hamamichi Y, Miyawaki T, Ono Y, Kamiya T, Akagi T, Hamada H, Hirose O, Isobe T, Yamada K, Kurotobi S, Mito H, Miyake T, Murakami Y, Nishi T, Shinohara M, Seguchi M, Tashiro S, Tomimatsu H. Clinical features of isolated noncompaction of the ventricular myocardium: long-term clinical course, hemodynamic properties, and genetic background. J Am Coll Cardiol. 1999;34:233–40.
7. Jenni R, Oechslin E, Schneider J, Attenhofer Jost C, Kaufmann PA. Echocardiographic and pathoanatomical characteristics of isolated left ventricular non-compaction: a step towards classification as a distinct cardiomyopathy. Heart. 2001;86:666–71.
8. Oechslin E, Jenni R. Left ventricular non-compaction revisited: a distinct phenotype with genetic heterogeneity? Eur Heart J. 2011;32:1446–56.
9. Aras D, Tufekcioglu O, Ergun K, Ozeke O, Yildiz A, Topaloglu S, Deveci B, Sahin O, Kisacik HL, Korkmaz S. Clinical features of isolated ventricular noncompaction in adults long-term clinical course, echocardiographic properties, and predictors of left ventricular failure. J Card Fail. 2006;12:726–33.
10. Habib G, Charron P, Eicher JC, Giorgi R, Donal E, Laperche T, Boulmier D, Pascal C, Logeart D, Jondeau G, Cohen-Solal A, Working Groups 'Heart Failure and Cardiomyopathies' and 'Echocardiography' of the French Society of Cardiology. Isolated left ventricular non-compaction in adults: clinical and echocardiographic features in 105 patients. Results from a French registry. Eur J Heart Fail. 2011;13:177–85.
11. Oechslin EN, Attenhofer Jost CH, Jenni R. Examination of isolated ventricular noncompaction (hypertrabeculation) as a distinct entity in adults. Am J Cardiol. 2012;109:776–7.

12. Wang C, Takasaki A, Watanabe Ozawa S, Nakaoka H, Okabe M, Miyao N, Saito K, Ibuki K, Hirono K, Yoshimura N, Yu X, Ichida F. Long-term prognosis of patients with left ventricular noncompaction- comparison between infantile and juvenile types. Circ J. 2017;81:694–700.
13. Towbin JA, Jefferies JL. Cardiomyopathies due to left ventricular noncompaction, mitochondrial and storage diseases, and inborn errors of metabolism. Circ Res. 2017;121:838–54.
14. Engberding R, Bender F. Identification of a rare congenital anomaly of the myocardium by two-dimensional echocardiography: persistence of isolated myocardial sinusoids. Am J Cardiol. 1984;53:1733–4.
15. Chin TK, Perloff JK, Williams RG, Jue K, Mohrmann R. Isolated noncompaction of left ventricular myocardium. A study of eight cases. Circulation. 1990;82:507–13.
16. Stollberger C, Finsterer J, Blazek G. Left ventricular hypertrabeculation/noncompaction and association with additional cardiac abnormalities and neuromuscular disorders. Am J Cardiol. 2002;90:899–902.
17. Arenas IA, Mihos CG, DeFaria Yeh D, Yucel E, Elmahdy HM, Santana O. Echocardiographic and clinical markers of left ventricular ejection fraction and moderate or greater systolic dysfunction in left ventricular noncompaction cardiomyopathy. Echocardiography. 2018;35(7):941–8.
18. Stollberger C, Gerger D, Jirak P, Wegner C, Finsterer J. Evolution of electrocardiographic abnormalities in association with neuromuscular disorders and survival in left ventricular hypertrabeculation/noncompaction. Ann Noninvasive Electrocardiol. 2014;19:567–73.
19. van Waning JI, Caliskan K, Hoedemaekers YM, van Spaendonck-Zwarts KY, Baas AF, Boekholdt SM, van Melle JP, Teske AJ, Asselbergs FW, Backx A, du Marchie Sarvaas GJ, Dalinghaus M, Breur J, Linschoten MPM, Verlooij LA, Kardys I, Dooijes D, Lekanne Deprez RH, AS IJ, van den Berg MP, Hofstra RMW, van Slegtenhorst MA, Jongbloed JDH, Majoor-Krakauer D. Genetics, clinical features, and long-term outcome of noncompaction cardiomyopathy. J Am Coll Cardiol. 2018;71:711–22.
20. Muser D, Nucifora G, Gianfagna E, Pavoni D, Rebellato L, Facchin D, Daleffe E, Proclemer A. Clinical spectrum of isolated left ventricular noncompaction: thromboembolic events, malignant left ventricular arrhythmias, and refractory heart failure. J Am Coll Cardiol. 2014;63:e39.
21. Tian T, Liu Y, Gao L, Wang J, Sun K, Zou Y, Wang L, Zhang L, Li Y, Xiao Y, Song L, Zhou X. Isolated left ventricular noncompaction: clinical profile and prognosis in 106 adult patients. Heart Vessel. 2013;29:645–52.
22. Stöllberger C, Blazek G, Gessner M, Bichler K, Wegner C, Finsterer J. Neuromuscular comorbidity, heart failure, and atrial fibrillation as prognostic factors in left ventricular hypertrabeculation/noncompaction. Herz. 2015;40:906–11.
23. Steffel J, Hürlimann D, Namdar M, Despotovic D, Kobza R, Wolber T, Holzmeister J, Haegeli L, Brunckhorst C, Lüscher TF, Jenni R, Duru F. Long-term follow-up of patients with isolated left ventricular noncompaction: role of electrocardiography in predicting poor outcome. Circ J. 2011;75:1728–34.
24. Stämpfli SF, Erhart L, Hagenbuch N, Stähli BE, Gruner C, Greutmann M, Niemann M, Kaufmann BA, Jenni R, Held L, Tanner FC. Prognostic power of NT-proBNP in left ventricular non-compaction cardiomyopathy. Int J Cardiol. 2017;236:321–7.
25. Asfalou I, Boulaamayl S, Raissouni M, Mouine N, Sabry M, Kheyi J, Doghmi N, Benyass A. Left ventricular noncompaction—a rare form of cardiomyopathy: revelation modes and predictors of mortality in adults through 23 cases. J Saudi Heart Assoc. 2017;29:102–9.
26. Lofiego C, Biagini E, Pasquale F, Ferlito M, Rocchi G, Perugini E, Bacchi-Reggiani L, Boriani G, Leone O, Caliskan K, ten Cate FJ, Picchio FM, Branzi A, Rapezzi C. Wide spectrum of presentation and variable outcomes of isolated left ventricular non-compaction. Heart. 2007;93:65–71.
27. Zuckerman WA, Richmond ME, Singh RK, Carroll SJ, Starc TJ, Addonizio LJ. Left-ventricular noncompaction in a pediatric population: predictors of survival. Pediatr Cardiol. 2011;32:406–12.
28. Shi WY, Moreno-Betancur M, Nugent AW, Cheung M, Colan S, Turner C, Sholler GF, Robertson T, Justo R, Bullock A, King I, Davis AM, Daubeney PEF, Weintraub RG, National Australian Childhood Cardiomyopathy Study. Long-term outcomes of childhood left ven-

tricular non-compaction cardiomyopathy: results from a national population-based study. Circulation. 2018;138(4):367–76.
29. Li S, Zhang C, Liu N, Bai H, Hou C, Wang J, Song L, Pu J. Genotype-positive status is associated with poor prognoses in patients with left ventricular noncompaction cardiomyopathy. Am Heart Assoc. 2018;7(20):e009910. https://doi.org/10.1161/JAHA.118.009910.
30. Andreini D, Pontone G, Bogaert J, Roghi A, Barison A, Schwitter J, Mushtaq S, Vovas G, Sormani P, Aquaro GD, Monney P, Segurini C, Guglielmo M, Conte E, Fusini L, Dello Russo A, Lombardi M, Gripari P, Baggiano A, Fiorentini C, Lombardi F, Bartorelli AL, Pepi M, Masci PG. Long-term prognostic value of cardiac magnetic resonance in left ventricle noncompaction: a prospective multicenter study. J Am Coll Cardiol. 2016;68:2166–81.
31. Peters F, Khandheria BK, Botha F, Libhaber E, Matioda H, Dos Santos C, Govender S, Meel R, Essop MR. Clinical outcomes in patients with isolated left ventricular noncompaction and heart failure. J Card Fail. 2014;20(10):709–15. https://doi.org/10.1016/j.cardfail.2014.07.007.
32. Kimura K, Takenaka K, Ebihara A, Uno K, Morita H, Nakajima T, Ozawa T, Aida I, Yonemochi Y, Higuchi S, Motoyoshi Y, Mikata T, Uchida I, Ishihara T, Komori T, Kitao R, Nagata T, Takeda S, Yatomi Y, Nagai R, Komuro I. Prognostic impact of left ventricular noncompaction in patients with Duchenne/Becker muscular dystrophy—prospective multicenter cohort study. Int J Cardiol. 2013;168(3):1900–4. https://doi.org/10.1016/j.ijcard.2012.12.058.
33. Greutmann M, Mah ML, Silversides CK, Klaassen S, Attenhofer Jost CH, Jenni R, Oechslin EN. Predictors of adverse outcome in adolescents and adults with isolated left ventricular noncompaction. Am J Cardiol. 2012;109:276–81.
34. Correia E, Rodrigues B, Santos L, Faria R, Ferreira P, Gama P, Nascimento C, Dionisio O, Cabral C, Santos O. Noncompaction of the ventricular myocardium: characterization and follow-up of an affected population. Rev Port Cardiol. 2011;30(3):323–31.
35. Brescia ST, Rossano JW, Pignatelli R, Jefferies JL, Price JF, Decker JA, Denfield SW, Dreyer WJ, Smith O, Towbin JA, Kim JJ. Mortality and sudden death in pediatric left ventricular noncompaction in a tertiary referral center. Circulation. 2013;127:2202–8.
36. Kofflard MJ, Waldstein DJ, Vos J, ten Cate FJ. Prognosis in hypertrophic cardiomyopathy observed in a large clinic population. Am J Cardiol. 1993;72:939–43.
37. Maron BJ, Casey SA, Poliac LC, Gohman TE, Almquist AK, Aeppli DM. Clinical course of hypertrophic cardiomyopathy in a regional United States cohort. JAMA. 1999;281:650–5.
38. Tian T, Yang Y, Zhou L, Luo F, Li Y, Fan P, Dong X, Liu Y, Cui J, Zhou X. Left ventricular non-compaction: a cardiomyopathy with acceptable prognosis in children. Heart Lung Circ. 2018;27(1):28–32. https://doi.org/10.1016/j.hlc.2017.01.013.
39. Czosek RJ, Spar DS, Khoury PR, Anderson JB, Wilmot I, Knilans TK, Jefferies JL. Outcomes, arrhythmic burden and ambulatory monitoring of pediatric patients with left ventricular noncompaction and preserved left ventricular function. Am J Cardiol. 2015;115(7):962–6. https://doi.org/10.1016/j.amjcard.2015.01.024.
40. Jefferies JL, Wilkinson JD, Sleeper LA, Colan SD, Lu M, Pahl E, Kantor PF, Everitt MD, Webber SA, Kaufman BD, Lamour JM, Canter CE, Hsu DT, Addonizio LJ, Lipshultz SE, Towbin JA, Investigators PCR. Cardiomyopathy phenotypes and outcomes for children with left ventricular myocardial noncompaction: results from the pediatric cardiomyopathy registry. J Card Fail. 2015;21(11):877–84. https://doi.org/10.1016/j.cardfail.2015.06.381.
41. Celiker A, Ozkutlu S, Dilber E, Karagöz T. Rhythm abnormalities in children with isolated ventricular noncompaction. Pacing Clin Electrophysiol. 2005;28(11):1198–202.
42. Wald R, Veldtman G, Golding F, Kirsh J, McCrindle B, Benson L. Determinants of outcome in isolated ventricular noncompaction in childhood. Am J Cardiol. 2004;94(12):1581–4.
43. Caliskan K, Kardos A, Szili-Torok T. Empty handed: a call for an international registry of risk stratification to reduce the 'sudden-ness' of death in patients with non-compaction cardiomyopathy. Europace. 2009;11:1138–9.

44. Marcus FI, McKenna WJ, Sherrill D, Basso C, Bauce B, Bluemke DA, Calkins H, Corrado D, Cox MG, Daubert JP, Fontaine G, Gear K, Hauer R, Nava A, Picard MH, Protonotarios N, Saffitz JE, Sanborn DM, Steinberg JS, Tandri H, Thiene G, Towbin JA, Tsatsopoulou A, Wichter T, Zareba W. Diagnosis of arrhythmogenic right ventricular cardiomyopathy/dysplasia: proposed modification of the Task Force Criteria. Eur Heart J. 2010;31:806–14.
45. Bhatia NL, Tajik AJ, Wilansky S, Steidley DE, Mookadam F. Isolated noncompaction of the left ventricular myocardium in adults: a systematic overview. J Card Fail. 2011;17:771–8.

Future Perspectives

10

Kadir Caliskan, Osama I. Soliman, and Folkert J. ten Cate

Noncompaction cardiomyopathy (NCCM) is genetically heterogeneous cardiomyopathy with a variable clinical presentation. The prognosis ranges from asymptomatic disease to severe, disabling, progressive heart failure.

However, the prevalence of NCCM is yet largely unknown. More definite answers are needed, based on molecular-biological, pathologic, clinical, and genetic analyses. Large international, multicenter prospective registries and expert consensus statements like in other cardiomyopathies are crucial to clarify current uncertainties. A clear patho anatomical / histo-pathological cut-off definition of NCCM should be the initial step towards a uniform imaging diagnosis and the differentiation from benign left ventricular noncompaction (LVNC) or secondary/acquired NCCM. The new classification should define the NCCM clearly as a separate disease entity, with its own nomenclature, classification, pathophysiology, and outcome.

Due to the genetic heterogeneity and lack of a clear view on the genotype-phenotype relationship of NCCM, routine genetic diagnostics, familial counseling, and cardiologic family screening should be encouraged. Current genetic testing reveals a relevant mutation in about one third only. Further molecular research is needed to investigate the role of additional, multiple mutations, and role in the phenotypic variability. Also, the perspective of new studies investigating modifying genetic effects or genome-environment interactions to explain the variability and age-dependent penetrance of this phenotype is challenging.

Different forms of the disease manifestations should be recognized: an isolated, mainly adult form of the disease, NCCM associated with congenital heart diseases (mainly in childhood) and NCCM in association with neuromuscular disease. Also,

K. Caliskan (✉) · F. J. ten Cate
Erasmus MC University Medical Center, Department of Cardiology,
Rotterdam, The Netherlands
e-mail: k.caliskan@erasmusmc.nl

O. I. Soliman
Erasmus MC University Medical Center, The Thoraxcenter, Rotterdam, The Netherlands

© Springer Nature Switzerland AG 2019
K. Caliskan et al. (eds.), *Noncompaction Cardiomyopathy*,
https://doi.org/10.1007/978-3-030-17720-1_10

benign LV and secondary noncompaction could be defined, especially in the athletes and (hypertensive) patient with African roots. The diagnostic clinical parameters should not only include the presence or absence of other concomitant cardiac diseases (congenital, valvular), the size, location and severity of excessive trabeculations, but also LV functional parameters (impaired LV function, rigid body rotation), RV involvement and dysfunction and possible genetic mutations. In this context, correctly defining the LV function is highly challenging, due to very irregular endocardial delineation. Therefore, routine LV ejection fraction measurements could be better refined, probabely with the newer imaging modalities like speckle tracking, global longitudinal systolic strain, and 3D echocardiography.

Risk stratification and prevention of sudden cardiac death (SCD) remains highly challenging, clinically needed. Strategies to improve the outcome of patients with this rare disease should come from large international multicenter registries, prospective randomized trials and registry-based studies to expand, confirm and refine the growing clinical experience of the last two decades.

This unique title will hopefully be a new landmark in our increasing knowledge of this yet rare, thus orphan disease!

Index

© Springer Nature Switzerland AG 2019
K. Caliskan et al. (eds.), *Noncompaction Cardiomyopathy*,
https://doi.org/10.1007/978-3-030-17720-1

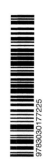